Probes for Health

J. Selwyn Crawford, K. W. Cross
P. R. Day, R. D. T. Farmer, Christine Hassall
E. G. Knox, T. Marshall, L. J. Opit
Susan Shaw, J. A. Stilwell

Edited by Gordon McLachlan

Published for the
Nuffield Provincial Hospitals Trust
by the Oxford University Press
London New York Toronto
1975

3 Prince Albert Road, London NW1 7SP
by Oxford University Press
Ely House, London W1
Glasgow New York Toronto Melbourne Wellington
Cape Town Salisbury Ibadan Nairobi Dar es Salaam Lusaka
Addis Ababa Bombay Calcutta Madras Karachi Lahore
Dacca Kuala Lumpur Singapore Hong Kong Tokyo

ISBN 0 19 721389 8

Designed by Bernard Crossland

Printed in Great Britain
by Burgess and Son (Abingdon) Ltd
Abingdon, Oxfordshire

Contents

Editorial

The problems of research even in these days of economic stringency are not confined to the restrictions arising from a shortage of financial backing. This particularly applies to health services research and development which is a relatively new concept which, as one seeks to move all the time towards a stronger definition of its elements, is shown to have all the multifaceted problems of the many disciplines and institutions concerned. It is also subject to the strains, stresses, and trials involved in the application of many disparate skills and techniques to the problems, some of them almost intractable to scientific inquiry, of essentially personal services where emotion tends to overwhelm reason.

The machinery of 'R and D' in itself is not the over-simple two-stroke function summed up by the idea of customer and contractor as peers. To achieve the effectiveness sought it must be a complex affair requiring understanding of human and institutional attitudes and motivations which are governed by conditions in which the NHS may not have any part at all and the reactions of the bureaucrats to which, without the leaven of understanding, may even be unsympathetic. Yet the fact that there is something labelled 'research' going on, is part these days of the necessary mechanism of social welfare administration and if it includes engagement in the necessary speculative thinking which is the preliminary to action for improvement so much the better, since it may even prove ultimately to be a necessary corrective to the occasional heedlessness of the not always co-ordinated drives of the machinery of government behind health services.

There is, however, nothing immaculate about the conception of research projects, and they need a supporting apparatus geared to the realities of the subject. The form such apparatus takes in the case of health services in the UK has still to be shaped effectively and the present are critical times in the education of those who are responsible for policy formation to what is involved over-all. The resources of manpower skills available are likely to be in short supply and the next few years are likely to be crucial to the forging and assembly of the several parts of the whole apparatus.

This poses the need for a theory to embrace the mechanisms and their effective functioning. Inevitably the universities will have a key role in any structure and its development. This volume gives some indication of what a unit based on a university outstanding in its attitude to and role in medical care can do, including the speculative thinking which is no indulgence but has an essential powerful drive of its own. It also gives some idea of the range of problems involved, the solution to which does not depend on the unit or university itself, but on the co-operation of the DHSS, the health authorities, and the academic community and on an awareness of the potential of such units on the part of all concerned with research.

Health services research and development is still a tender plant which needs special cultivation if it is to grow and contribute to the improvement of health services at all operational levels and so of health generally; and public policies towards its sponsorship, financing and management must reflect this requirement.

GORDON MCLACHLAN

3 Prince Albert Road,
London NW1
April 1975

E. G. Knox
MD, FRCP, FFCM
Health Services Research Centre
Department of Social Medicine
University of Birmingham

Research and health services

Research and health services

This book arises from an invitation by the Nuffield Provincial Hospitals Trust to assemble an exposition of work carried out at Birmingham in the field of health services research. It was not an easy invitation to accept. Health services research is often an *ad hoc* process and its content at any one time reflects responses to a variety of contemporary pressures and opportunities, as well as to specific requests from service authorities. Much of it is 'topical', if not necessarily ephemeral, and it is difficult to hold back items of completed work to await the completion of others, in order to assemble them together in a book. It is equally difficult to bend consecutive scientific studies towards an exposition of a common subject, a common technique, or a common purpose, and it would be a remarkable coincidence if they fell naturally within such a coherent theme. Nevertheless, the invitation was accepted for two main reasons.

First, the Birmingham Health Services Research Centre was built with funds provided by the Nuffield Provincial Hospitals Trust, the idea sprang from a series of studies promoted by the Trust, and although the major source of funds following its opening in 1972 have come from the DHSS, the Trust has continued to support work carried out in the unit. If the Trust has paternal feelings towards us we welcome them, and would like to commemorate its interest, and its energetic and pioneering promotional activities in this field.

Second, although health services research is no longer a new idea—several units dedicated to its purposes have been set up in this country and elsewhere, there is also a journal devoted to the subject, and recent expositions of its content already exist (see refs. 1, 3, 4, 5, 6)—it might be valuable to show how the subject looks from the point of view of the workers in a single unit. A rapidly developing field of work, interacting with a changing administrative context (especially in the UK) and a changing research technology, makes it attractive to try and capture and display its content and approaches at a particular place and at a particular point in time. A contemporary impression of this kind may even have some historical value when the discipline eventually settles down to be a routine activity—or is finally suppressed.

The untidiness and variability displayed by a consecutive sample of studies might serve indeed to emphasize the problem-orientated nature of the job. Perhaps the varying approaches could serve to demonstrate the wide and widening range of techniques involved, and to dissuade others from the notion that health services research is no more than a special application of epidemiology. The book might also supply a platform for saying fairly precisely what the workers in a particular unit think the subject is about.

THE APPLICATIONS AND APPLICABILITY OF HEALTH
SERVICES RESEARCH

Health services research is applied research and it is wasted if it is not applied. It is necessary from the outset of a study, even for its good design, to ascertain that the results can in fact be applied, and to elicit some assurance that they might be. The appropriate people, the necessary powers, and the administrative pathways of application should preferably be identified before the research begins, and there is seldom any value in providing solutions to questions or to decision dilemmas which have never yet arisen and which are unlikely to do so. Occasionally, we may envisage the need for an administrative mechanism which does not yet exist, and we may design research whose results may call that mechanism into being; but this is only to admit that our objectives have been oblique, and does not infringe basic principles.

Cherns (2) and others have pointed out that research activities span a range whose extremes extend from inquiries with highly general but remotely applicable conclusions to those which are local, topical, and possibly ephemeral, but in which the intention to apply the results is so immediate as to constitute an explicit part of the research plan. He calls this kind of research 'action research' and in so far as his analysis is valid, much health services research lies well towards the 'action research' end of the spectrum. However, the notion of 'action research' and a devotion to application, have sometimes been carried to the point where a programme is all action and no research. Indeed the virtues of involvement have sometimes been regarded as an excuse for absent results and even for absent research objectives. Simple innovations designed without reference to the furtherance of knowledge, are sometimes described in these circumstances as 'experiments', although the notion that there may be questions to be answered somehow gets lost.

Innovation and change without question or answer is an approach foreign to a valid philosophy of health services research. Research is always a question of and a quest for knowledge; it encompasses questions of *how*, as well as questions of *what*, and the research and its environment may be highly interactive, but it *always* involves questions and its purpose is to seek answers. 'Experiments' without research objectives cannot be recognized as research.

The outcome of successfully designed and executed research into health services is change, and the purpose of the change (and of the research) is the benefit of the users of the service. This, of course, is a common objective of all those engaged in the health service, but in the local contexts in which decisions are made it becomes one among a group of aims. They may include professional, political, legal, educational, and economic objectives, and it would be foolish to assume that conflicts could never arise. It would be equally foolish to assume that all research, all questions, and all answers, will be welcome all of the time to everyone engaged in the service.

Indeed they are not, and the discipline of asking explicit questions about health service policies and implementations in a manner which permits and provides exact answers, can be seen as frankly threatening. The reformulation of a confused or rhetorical question in a manner which might lead to an exact answer based on evidence, may sometimes render the query itself unaskable. Research workers whose plans have been frustrated sometimes take consolation in the thought that at least they must have formulated an important and pertinent question.

Research may also be a frank nuisance to health service administrators who want information which will make their decisions easier, and are offered only that which might make their decisions better. Health services research workers come to recognize this difference sharply and to balance their programmes to provide an acceptable balance between research which can be seen as helpful and that which might be seen as needling.

The pattern of health services research development in a particular context, and its subsequent applicability, depend crucially on the power-structure of the service. There is nothing to be gained by being mealy-mouthed about the notion of power; it provides the necessary outlet for health services research and it determines the pattern of work undertaken. If in particular circumstances there is no central control of the total financial allocations to a service or of the manner of deploying resources, and no hope of obtaining such control, there is little value in research whose outlets depend upon such control. If a central administration has no means of influencing the way in which its practitioners behave (for example in terms of their geographical distribution or their prescribing habits) then there is no immediate value in providing data which would give guidance on such behaviour, if the power to change it existed.

The administrative power structure will also determine the range of techniques which a health services research unit might apply. An administration which largely rejects scientific studies of its own activities will effectively limit research to 'observational' work, and the scientists may tend to concentrate upon investigations designed to demonstrate the defects of the system. The methodology will be very close to that of classical observational epidemiology. An administration which prefers interested research workers to be integrated into the service rather than excluded from it, will encourage the development of techniques applicable in planning and in implementation as well as in *post hoc* evaluation. The broadest range of research will be developed when research is promoted, encouraged, and assisted in relation to the whole of the evaluation/planning/control cycle. In these circumstances, health services research becomes concerned comprehensively with observation, prediction, experiment, control, and the setting of operational standards and objectives.

THE TECHNIQUES OF HEALTH SERVICES RESEARCH
The administrative integration (or otherwise) of health services research determines the range of methods to be deployed, and at its most effective its activities extend into every part of a cybernetic planning cycle.

At each level of an organization this cycle may be seen as starting with the setting of objectives in the light of external constraints. Health objectives are to be preferred, but in the absence of exact knowledge of the effect of health care services upon health, they may have to be set mainly in terms of the delivery of items of care such as consultations, operations, or days in hospital. It is necessary, at all events, that objectives are set in terms of verbs of visible action, so called 'behavioural' objectives, so that subsequent evidence of having met objectives can be sought. Without such objectives, subsequent evaluation of the outcome is precluded. Methods of achieving the objectives may then be postulated and a choice made between them. This is followed by implementation. The next step, evaluating outcomes, leads to modification of the techniques of implementation, or to changes in objectives, or the way in which they are stated, or to attempts to release the situation from external constraints. The process is continuous, contains many internal loops, and is itself contained within larger cycles.

Health services research finds a place in each of these component activities. It is concerned globally in the formulation of objectives in terms whose outcome can be measured, in the evaluation of outcomes and in the re-formulation of objectives in the light of results, or of difficulties in measuring them. In less global terms it is concerned also in the planning and execution of service experiments, in the design of intelligence and information systems used for the control of experimental and definitive services, in research upon the processes of implementation, in social/administrative inquiries into the process of decision-making and the formulation of policies, and in the prior evaluation of proposals through simulation and mathematical modelling techniques. The repertoire of method includes epidemiology and statistics in the traditional sense, operational research, work study, behavioural research, economic studies, electronic data processing, systems analysis and design, retrospective and prospective observational studies, randomized trials and computer simulation. The outcomes of these research activities include statistical digests and reviews of service, statistical tests of hypotheses, the identification of defects in existing services, conditional predictions of the consequences of different decisions, specifications of developed information systems, economic evaluations and predictions, the consequences of different manpower and staffing policies, draft standards of practice, and so on. As remarked at the beginning, this goes far beyond the range of 'epidemiology' as it is often understood. A fully developed research programme does not concede containment to any particular segment of the cycle.

It would be difficult, however, to guess at the balance of activities required of this discipline in any given context, and especially in the

UK following the recent reorganization of the NHS. One may hazard that the chief requirement of the central authorities (for example, the DHSS) will be related to questions of long-range policy and planning, and operations relating to large-scale innovations (such as cancer-screening programmes) where a degree of national uniformity could be envisaged. The regional health authorities will presumably need information to guide them on questions of capital expenditure, and on medical- and nursing-manpower planning and deployment. The regional and area health authorities will both be concerned to identify defects in existing services and to devise methods of overcoming them. All parties, including district management teams, health care planning teams, health service research workers and clinicians, will require the development of intelligence-processing and care-scheduling information systems. Thus, a different balance of techniques may be required for servicing different levels of the health care administration with economic, theoretical, and simulation studies, and studies of the over-all effectiveness of service policies predominating at a central level, and with field-study-based evaluations of efficient delivery of care predominating at local levels. However, over-all trends in health care research at every level will depend upon the way in which the need for and acceptability of hard evidence develops in the different loci. The tune will be called by the customers.

So far as the papers in this book are concerned, we would ask only that the balance is treated as accidental and without particular significance; it is virtually a random sample, and too small for drawing conclusions. The list of publications from the Centre at the end of the book is added in order to ameliorate the problem of sample size, but even this reflects no more than an initial foray at a time of rapid change. For the time being, and probably for the foreseeable future, only the broadest technical base is sufficient.

This broad technical base is required not only by those engaged in whole-time research but by those who chiefly use its results, that is, members of health care authorities and the medical and non-medical administrators who are responsible for the coherence and effectiveness of health services. It is necessary therefore that their specialist education is based upon the same techniques. It follows that workers in health services research must play a major part in training recruits to the administrative branch of the service and in the continuing education of those already in post. It is not suggested that all health services research units must do this, or that they must all be situated within universities but that an integrated approach and a joint use of resources is a *sine qua non* of these activities.

THE ADMINISTRATIVE CONTEXT OF HEALTH SERVICES RESEARCH

The first corollary of a wide range of necessary skills is that a reasonably comprehensive research programme cannot be carried out by any single class of worker. It requires a research team of a certain minimum size which should contain non-medical as well as medical scientists. This minimum scientific 'critical mass' must consist mainly of experienced people with reasonably long-term expectations of employment. Junior and trainee staff, and workers on short-time or 'visiting' contracts must be considered supernumerary for this purpose. It is difficult to put actual numbers to these notions, but four or five senior research workers including at least two medical scientists is probably the effective minimum for mounting a substantial programme of work with some assurance of continuity. This would be appropriate in a situation where the unit is attached to, or is part of, an existing academic department of social or community medicine, or an MRC unit, and where part of the 'critical mass' and 'continuity' requirement is supplied from this source and through contacts with other academic or scientific departments.

A number of short-term or part-time posts may also be provided, but there cannot be too many of them. This is a field in which a great deal of negotiation is required, where mistakes or unfinished work are very damaging, and where it is difficult for a whole-time worker to supervise more than one or two juniors in the course of his work. The core staff and the shorter-term workers will also need the technical support of secretarial and medical staff, programmers and technicians, the use of computer and data-processing facilities and the (part-time) services of an administrator. Altogether a unit consisting of 12 to 20 people, occupying a floor space of 500 m² (including storage, technical, and teaching space) and requiring a budget of £70,000–150,000 per annum may be envisaged. These figures are quite arbitrary, depend on the assumption of an existing academic or other research base, and are clearly subject to wide possible variations, but they are given in order to provide a concrete basis for the notion of a research unit. A unit without a supporting base would need to be considerably larger in order to protect its projects, and even its existence, against stochastic extinction as a result of changing staffs.

The apposition of health services research units with existing departments of social and community medicine is enforcing a welcome clarification of the purposes and techniques of such departments. Social medicine has often been described, loosely, as consisting jointly of health services research on the one hand, and epidemiology on the other. This was an unsatisfactory division on logical and syntactical grounds in that it contrasted an outlet with a technique. A more satisfactory and explicit description would counterpoint the health services studies with studies of the aetiologies of disease, and specifically, since the major determinants of health are here, with the effects of the environment. Other components of the subject can no doubt be recognized but these two, health care studies and studies of the environmental determinants of health and disease, are overriding. The subject depends upon them for its integrity and cannot properly be pursued without a major interest in both. More urgent than these conceptual reappraisals and reformulations, however, is the search for an adequate framework within which an enhancement of these activities can be pursued.

The choice of a suitable administrative mechanism for a research centre is determined by the need for a cybernetic relationship at each level between health services administrators and health services research workers, rather than 'ownership' of one by the other. In a layered structure such as the NHS it is probably best if at each level the administrative and research workers obtain their resources from a common source, rather than the research team should depend for its finances and staff establishment upon the administrative bodies whose decisions it may service. This is not to say that an NHS authority should not sponsor and finance the marginal costs of research carried out at its request, but there is a basic necessity to develop and secure the research resource on which such activities can take place.

The need for administrative separation is one side of the coin; the need for operational integration is the other. The result is a pattern of activities based upon a contract between three parties (if such a contract is possible: a benevolent conspiracy if it is not).

The administrative requirements in turn raise a number of issues relating to the appointment of scientific staffs. The most difficult and urgent at the present time relate to career structures and job security. This is especially so in a unit (such as Birmingham) where a university is acting as the agent through which the research workers are employed and housed, where the funds are mainly derived from a central authority (DHSS) and where the staff of the unit have working affiliations with regional and area health authorities, as well as with the DHSS. As far as medical scientists are concerned the problems are of two kinds, one relating to joint appointments between university and health authorities and the second relating to the terms of appointment of 'core' staffs in research units. The solution of the first is technically easy and we can hope, even anticipate, that arrangements already arrived at in some areas will eventually be achieved in all. It is simply a question of providing satisfactory arrangements for honorary cross appointments between academic and services staff in a manner established for many years in clinical academic units. The solution of the second problem is more difficult, but vital.

The issue here is whether (or rather when) a mechanism can be formulated which permits the establishment of career posts in sufficient numbers for 'core' appointments in research centres. At present very few workers have 'tenure' and this state of affairs is largely limited to university staffs (for example directors of units) who were in post when the centres were established and who are not dependent for their job security or career promotion upon the contracts which they negotiate. There is little in the terms of appointments of other 'core' posts to attract senior workers or to retain experienced ones. Second-class status is unlikely to commend itself to first-class people, nor even to directors who find themselves unable to undertake long-term or other substantial commitments on behalf of their units.

The problems of non-medical staffs are less acute from the point of view of the viability of research units, although no less so from the points of view of the workers themselves, and these problems will also have to be solved.

Together, these problems and their apparently tardy solutions are coming to represent, for some workers, a question of faith. The issue, for them, is whether health services research is to be developed and supported vigorously as something that is here to stay and is a necessary and integral part of a health care delivery system: or whether it is to remain a subject for ambivalence, to be supported half-heartedly, and its practitioners excluded from first-class citizenship in the vague hope (and practical certainty) that they might eventually go away.

References

1. 'Research in medical care', *Br. med. Bull.* **30,** no. 3 (1974).
2. CHERNS, A. (1969). 'Social research and its diffusion', *Human Relations,* **22,** 209–18.
3. MCLACHLAN, G. (ed.) (1975). *Measuring for Management* (Oxford University Press for the Nuffield Provincial Hospitals Trust).
4. —— (1971). *Portfolio for Health, Problems and Progress in Medical Care,* Sixth Series (Oxford University Press for the Nuffield Provincial Hospitals Trust).
5. —— (1973). *Portfolio for Health 2, Problems and Progress in Medical Care,* Eighth Series (Oxford University Press for the Nuffield Provincial Hospitals Trust).
6. —— (1974). *Positions, Movements, and Directions in Health Services Research* (Oxford University Press for the Nuffield Provincial Hospitals Trust).

E. G. Knox
MD, FRCP, FFCM
Health Services Research Centre
Department of Social Medicine
University of Birmingham

Simulation studies of breast cancer screening programmes

Simulation studies of breast cancer screening programmes

The screening procedures available for detecting early breast cancer include palpation by doctor or nurse, the teaching of self-palpation, mammography (soft tissue X-rays), xeroradiography (use of xerograph plates instead of photographic film), infra-red photography using reflected radiation, thermography (scanning the intensity of emitted infra-red radiation), and the estimation of urinary steroids.

The urinary steroid test is different from the others in that it is aimed towards distinguishing high-risk from low-risk groups of women, rather than the direct detection of existing tumours. It needs only to be performed once and its purpose is the prescription of different subsequent regimes of surveillance for the two groups, including the possibility of non-surveillance for the low-risk group. Unfortunately, this purpose is complicated by the fact that a positive urinary steroid test is also associated with a poor prognosis in women who have cancer, and limitation of surveillance to the high-risk group will not necessarily detect those with the greatest prospect of benefit from early treatment. The questions surrounding this issue have yet to be answered.

Thermography and infra-red photography are neither very sensitive nor very specific and produce substantial numbers of false positives. They are certainly time-consuming, and their chief application may be as diagnostic aids in women already known to have a breast abnormality (1, 2, 3).

Mammography and palpation by a doctor are the only screening procedures so far subjected to large-scale randomized clinical trials. The Health Insurance Plan (HIP) study in New York (4) suggested that each alone had poor sensitivity, and the combination only moderate sensitivity, but that their joint application succeeded in detecting cancers at relatively early stages, and reduced the mortality from breast cancer during a subsequent period of investigation.

Presumably the sensitivity of such a regime could be improved by carrying out investigations more frequently, and the total yield could be increased by extending the process beyond the four years of the HIP investigations. However, improved results would be bought at a cost which would go beyond the necessary increased investment, and would include a large number of extra biopsies. There were about twenty biopsies for every death saved or postponed in the HIP study group. Not all of them can be regarded as *extra* biopsies because biopsies also took place in the control group, although it is not possible from the published data to ascertain how many. In addition to extra biopsies, say 10 per death saved, mammography incurs a risk of inducing cancer in women who would not otherwise have had the disease. General estimates for the risk of whole body radiation are currently accepted at about 200 cases, per million exposed, per rad of exposure (5). Mammography cannot be regarded as equivalent to whole body radiation, but the breast and adjacent haemopoietic tissues are sites with high tumour frequencies and a thousand women, each exposed on ten occasions to a recently typical 5 rad per examination, will probably generate between one and three iatrogenic cases of cancer. (The basis of this statement will be developed later.) Approximately 40 women in every 1,000 in the general population will die from breast cancer, and a crude extrapolation from the HIP study to a 10-exposure regime would suggest a saving of about five lives. At first sight, the potential benefits appear not *very* much greater than the potential hazards.

Moreover, the balance might change as a screening service was extended. The effect of a small to moderate investment in breast cancer screening would almost certainly be a net numerical benefit, particularly if radiation exposure were reduced or limited to older age-groups, and even the lives lost would be twenty years or so older than the lives saved. With increasing investment, however, we might expect a diminishing return on the one hand and a linear accumulation of hazard on the other, together with a resultant extension into younger age-groups with lower yields and higher risks of damage.

The issues surrounding the conversion of procedures to services are quantitative and the outcomes depend crucially upon estimates of the relative effectiveness of early treatment, a matter which was in doubt until the HIP study was reported. Within five years of registration, the study group had a mortality about one-third better than the controls, and provisional figures for seven years of follow-up suggest that this ratio has been maintained. It is important however not to misinterpret relative mortalities such as these, or to extrapolate them directly to the context of an extended screening programme with long-term follow-up. For example, the study group savings represented only 13 per cent of all the breast cancers discovered during the four-year screening programme. This proportion might increase or decrease as follow-up proceeds, but because many of the anticipated deaths in the control group had already occurred by seven years, the gap between the two groups is more likely to narrow than to widen.

It must be remembered in addition that the 30,000 women in the HIP study group could be expected throughout their lifetimes to generate about 2,000 breast cancers with about 1,200 deaths and that the seven-year saving of 38 cases (6) (that is, the difference between the study group and the control group) will represent only about 3 per cent of all these deaths. It follows that any proposals for an effective screening service must involve extrapolations far beyond the range of the HIP testbed.

This paper is concerned with the process of extrapolation. Almost all the facts on which an accurate projection might be based are subject to a range of uncertainty against which we have to place a wide range of policy alternatives. What tests, how many of each, which ages, in what sequence? The purposes of the extrapolation are to determine the best and worst which could reasonably be expected for each proposal set against each combination of factual uncertainties; and if possible to determine in advance the important questions which will arise and will need to be answered as a programme is developed and extended.

Methods

The exercise which follows is a particular usage of a generalized computer program described in detail elsewhere (7), and capable of being adapted to a particular population context and to a particular health problem through the provision of a statement of the normal (female) life-table and a list of the names of the pathological states which will be recognized within the population. A statement of the natural history of the disease process must then be provided in the form of a 'transition matrix' which gives estimated transfer rates between the various pathological states, modified suitably according to the age of the woman or the duration of the state. This set of values is adjusted iteratively until an output is produced which matches available data on incidence, prevalence, and mortality. If, as sometimes happens, more than one natural history statement is capable of mimicking these facts, then the natural history will have to be treated as one of the uncertainties. Subsequent runs will then have to be repeated for a range of natural history alternatives, and each prediction of results will be conditional upon the accuracy of the natural history used. Changes in natural history consequent upon treatment must also be declared and again adjusted iteratively to fit available case-fatality data. The computer program is now in a position to manipulate a complete life to death process in a single cohort of subjects.

At this point it is possible to add details of the screening procedures to be considered, specifying the clinico-pathological states to which they are to be applied, their sensitivities or specificities in relation to each, and the transfers which will occur following detection or non-detection. Finally, the ages at which the tests are to be offered are listed, together with anticipated attendance rates at each age.

The policy alternatives are usually arranged in incremental series and the results compared with each other and with the results of providing no service at all. The outputs thus permit appraisals of benefits and costs in absolute and in marginal terms.

For the purposes of the present exercise, some of the entries to the simulation programme remained fixed throughout and will be described here under 'Methods'. The entries derived through iterative fitting of outputs to available data, and the consequences of alternative-policy extrapolations, will be described later under 'Results'. The fixed entries were as follows:

(a) Life-table. Mortality from all causes was specified as the female life-table for England and Wales supplied by the Registrar General. This governs transfers from NORMAL, and from all other living states, to DEAD FROM OTHER CAUSE.

(b) List of pathological states. Transfers from NORMAL to DEAD OF THIS DISEASE were accomplished through a series of intermediate states namely PRE-CLINICAL (ie non-self-detectable), EARLY CLINICAL (ie potentially self-detectable), and LATE CLINICAL, CANCERS. For each of these there was assigned a corresponding 'TREATED' state, and each of the resulting six classes of cancer was resolved into a 'HIGH GRADE' and a 'LOW GRADE' variety.

It was necessary for some runs to resolve NORMAL into HIGH RISK NORMAL and LOW RISK NORMAL; also, BIOPSIED NORMAL. It was necessary also to resolve each grade of untreated PRE-CLINICAL CANCER according to post-examination status, namely PALPATION POSITIVE, PALPATION NEGATIVE, MAMMOGRAM POSITIVE, and MAMMO-GRAM NEGATIVE.

The full set for the simulation exercise included twenty-six defined states and it was convenient to list them at the outset and keep them constant throughout, although the subsequent transition matrices did not use every state at every run.

Although the values of transfer rates were defined iteratively, and are described later, the general sequence of the transfer-pattern was held constant. Thus, normal passed to pre-clinical, to early clinical, and thence to late clinical with no skipping and no reversals. Grades were established at the first transfer and once determined, remained constant throughout and followed separate natural histories without interconversion. Each of the untreated states could 'branch' to its treated state, the pre-clinicals only through screening procedures and the others either through screening or through spontaneous presenta-tion. Every pathological state, treated or untreated, was assigned a mortality; only the four types of 'normal' were exempted from special mortalities over and above the life-table mortalities.

Results

The development of the simulation took place in four main stages, although there was some recursive interaction between them. The steps were (i) development of a natural history specification capable of explaining available incidence, prevalence, mortality, and case-fatality data; (ii) development of palpation and mammography screening specifications, particularly sensitivities and specificities capable of explaining and mimicking the results of the HIP experi-ment; (iii) extrapolation from adequate mimicry of the HIP experi-ment, to predicting the results of extended screening services; and (iv) examination of the scope of urinary-steroid 'pre-screening' tests.

The main recursive interaction between the stages occurred when it was found that in order to reproduce so quick an effect upon mortality as that actually observed in New York, it was necessary to specify a more rapid progression of the pre-clinical and early clinical lesions than had previously been envisaged. The first two stages thus ran through several interleaved adjustments before progression to the last two stages was possible.

THE NATURAL HISTORY

(a) Onsets

The natural history finally adopted comprised forty-six main transitions. The basic primary step was a transition from normal to pre-clinical cancer of which half the transfers were to high grade, and half to low grade.

This 50:50 division was used consistently for the later parts of the study, following some initial attempts to manipulate the ratio according to age, and so reflect the observed age-variation of prognosis. However, the manipulations were cumbersome and time-consuming, and although they proved capable of altering natural prognosis in the manner intended, they did not at subsequent stages successfully mimic the observed age-dependence of the effectiveness of screening. The HIP trial seemed to indicate that screening was effective in saving lives only after the age of 50 years. Detailed manipulations of the high-grade:low-grade ratio were therefore abandoned, with the alternative conclusions that the mimicry of such fine detail was beyond the capacity of the simulation system as it stands at present, or that the HIP age-dependence effect might be a sampling artefact dependent on small numbers.

The arbitrary 50:50 division between high-grade and low-grade onsets may be justified simply as a question of definition; as used in this simulation study the terms refer simply to the worst half and to the best half. It must be emphasized that the classification bears no direct relationship to histological gradings, which in any case are usually expressed on a three-point scale.

The age-specific onset-rates finally adopted are given in Table 1, where they can be compared with registration-rates for clinical cancer in one part of the USA (Connecticut) and one part of the UK (Birmingham) (8). The data are not to be compared exactly with the values adopted for simulation since they represent different stages of the process, and as might be anticipated the simulated values are higher than the observations at early ages, and somewhat lower at later ages. It must be recalled also, that the simulation values refer to a single cohort, while the observations are cross-sectional. (The elevated simulation value adopted in the earliest age-group was designed to 'catch-up' with occurrences before age 30, the starting age for the simulation.)

TABLE 1

Simulated age-specific onset rates for pre-clinical cancer, compared with registration rates in Connecticut and Birmingham (1963–6) (Rates are percentage per annum)

				Age			
	30–34	−39	−49	−59	−69	−79	80+
Simulation	0·08	0·05	0·16	0·21	0·23	0·22	0·20
Connecticut	0·02	0·06	0·14	0·17	0·20	0·28	0·33
Birmingham	0·02	0·05	0·11	0·14	0·17	0·20	0·26

The simulated onset rates began as guesses which were subsequently adjusted and readjusted until the cumulative age-specific incidence of clinical carcinoma put out by the simulation system matched in general form that reported in Great Britain as a whole (9). However, these figures were subsequently modified in order to raise the total incidence to a point about midway between British and American observations. This was a compromise, and there were two main reasons for it. The first was that realistic second-stage adjustments depended largely upon matching American (HIP) results. The second was that a 'mid-Atlantic' position probably represents fairly closely the situation for which we should now be planning in Britain. Changes in reproductive patterns in Britain, as elsewhere, seem likely to bring the British experience of breast cancer towards the higher levels already observed in the USA.

In the event, the compromise gave accumulated onsets for clinical carcinoma 19 per cent in excess of the 1966 registrations for England and Wales. By comparison the Connecticut accumulated data for 1963–6 were 28 per cent in excess of the accumulated Birmingham registrations for that period. The simulation gave a final case fatality of 64·6 per cent compared with 66·2 per cent for England and Wales: obtained by comparing deaths in 1971 with registrations five years previously (10, 11). Details of the comparisons are given in Table 2.

(b) Onward transfers

Onward transfer rates, from pre-clinical cancer through more advanced stages, were designed in order to produce an age-specific distribution of deaths similar to that observed in England and Wales, together with an equivalent final case-fatality. However, a range of different rates of progress proved equally capable of achieving this end and the choice depended mainly on a later stage of the iteration, namely the fitting of outputs to the results of the HIP study. This

TABLE 2

Deaths (1971) and registrations (1966) in England and Wales, compared with outputs of simulation

| | Age | | | | | | | |
	−29	−39	−49	−59	−69	−79	−95	*Total*
England and Wales 1966 registrations	105	915	3,248	4,163	4,250	2,900	1,320	16,901
Accumulated registrations reduced*	4	37	153	302	455	559	606	
Accumulated simulated clinical cancers	0	56	192	368	540	663	722	
England and Wales 1971 deaths	30	308	1,322	2,390	3,040	2,490	1,602	11,182
Accumulated deaths reduced*	1	12	60	154	254	343	401	
Accumulated simulated deaths	0	19	81	189	315	413	460	

*Reduced figures were obtained by applying to the accumulated previous row, the fraction 10,000/278,903, being the ratio between deaths from all causes in the simulated cohort and among females in England and Wales in 1971.

process will be described later but a selection of outcomes of the adopted plan are presented in the second half of Table 2, and its essential elements were as follows.

First, high rates of transfer were assigned from pre-clinical to early-clinical cancer. For high-grade cancer the transfer rate was set at 70 per cent per annum (compound) for the first two years, falling thereafter to 40 per cent per annum, and after another four years to 20 per cent per annum, to allow for a small hypothetical residuum of slow-growing tumours (12, 13, 14). For low-grade cancers the corresponding rates were 40, 30, and 16 per cent. The resulting cumulative decay rates are quite rapid and three years from onset, for example, only 25 per cent of low-grade tumours would still be in the pre-clinical stage, and only 5 per cent of the high-grade tumours.

Rapid onward transfers were also ascribed to early clinical cancers, with changes either to late clinical cancer or to treated early cancer. For high-grade tumours the first transfer proceeded at 50 per cent per annum for two years rising subsequently to 80 per cent for four years and falling again thereafter. Low-grade cancers proceeded at half these rates. Spontaneous presentation for treatment was at 70 per cent per annum, initially, for the high-grade tumours, and 50 per cent for the low grades. Spontaneous presentations of late clinical cancers were set at the same values, grade for grade, as in the early clinical cancers.

Every clinical and pre-clinical stage of cancer was assigned a fatality rate. This applied also to classes attained only through screening procedures and was necessary in order to avoid an artefactual benefit of screening simply through transfer to a class with no mortality rate allocated. Each untreated stage was allocated a mortality rate higher than the earlier stage, and high-grade cancers were allocated rates greater than low-grade cancers. The general pattern was represented by a moderate rate in the first year rising to higher rates over the next few years and a subsequent fall, the peak rates being set somewhat earlier for the advanced and high-grade cancers than for the early and low-grade cancers. Thus, untreated high-grade late clinical cancers died at 16 per cent per annum in the first year, 32 per cent per annum compound in the next three years, falling to 16 and later still to 8 per cent. Low-grade equivalents died at three-quarters of these rates. Treated high-grade late cancer was allocated the same mortality as late untreated low-grade; late treated low-grade had two-thirds of this mortality. Treated early high-grade had the same mortality as late untreated low-grade; treated early low-grade had two-thirds of this mortality.

Although the annual mortality rates were thus set in a modal distribution, the cumulative survival curves descended in a pattern resembling a modified negative exponential decay. A summary of the different survival curves for the main classes of cancer, provided they did not die of another cause, is given in Table 3. The results compare reasonably, for example, with large-scale follow-up data reported by Bloom (15). Bloom's ten-year survival for stage 3 low-grade cancers was 44 per cent, corresponding with a simulated 37 per cent for late-treated low-grade. His stage 1 low-grade survival after ten years was 61 per cent, compared with a simulated 50 per cent for treated early clinical and 69 per cent for treated pre-clinical.

Bloom's stage 3 high-grade cancers had a 10 per cent survival at ten years, a figure which compared reasonably accurately with the simulated 9 per cent for untreated late cancer, but less accurately with treated late cancer; in this respect simulated fatalities were rather optimistic. Stage 1 high-grade survivals were 52 per cent, compared with a simulated 57 per cent for treated pre-clinicals and a simulated 37 per cent for treated early clinical cancers; the simulation is a little pessimistic here.

TABLE 3

Simulated percentage survivals in successive years from cancers of different kinds

	Years of follow-up						
	0	*1*	*2*	*3*	*4*	*6*	*10*
High-grade cancers							
Untreated late	100	84	57	39	26	19	9
Treated late	100	88	67	58	49	38	23
Treated early	100	92	77	73	61	52	37
Treated pre-clinical	100	100	94	89	83	73	57
Low-grade cancers							
Untreated late	100	88	67	58	49	38	23
Treated late	100	92	77	73	61	52	37
Treated early	100	94	83	73	68	60	50
Treated pre-clinical	100	100	96	92	88	82	69

MIMICRY OF HIP RESULTS

(a) *HIP findings*

The HIP experiment used a control and a study group, each of 31,000 women. Only 20,200 of the study group actually attended for screening, and with further drop-outs an average of only 16,300 attended each of the four tests offered. For comparison, the simulated cohort consisted of 10,000 female births of whom 9,170 were still alive, without clinical cancer, at 50 years. Therefore, the benefits measured in the HIP experiment must be reduced in the ratio 9,170/16,300 (ie $\times 0.563$) in order to estimate the benefits to be mimicked in the simulation. After five years of follow-up from the point of entry to the HIP study, there were 23 fewer deaths in the study group than in the controls, and after seven years, 38. In the simulation we therefore need to adjust the parameters of four successive annual tests around age 50, until they produce respective savings of about 13, and about 21 breast cancer deaths after the same periods of time.

(b) *Sensitivity and specificity*

The main adjustable parameters of the simulated screening procedures are the separate sensitivities and specificities of mammography and of palpation. The sensitivities affect importantly the numbers of cancers detected and the numbers of deaths saved;

specificities, on the other hand, chiefly affect the number of biopsied normals; that is, the number of biopsied non-cancers who would otherwise not have received a biopsy. The allocation of the sensitivity parameters, and the allocation of the onward transfer values for pre-clinical cancers, are interactive, because, when we apply a sensitivity of x per cent, we have to ask 'x per cent of what?'

In one sense, the allocated sensitivity value is a partial definition of what we mean by 'pre-clinical', and of the stage in the disease process where 'potential detectability' is deemed to begin. In cases such as this, where there is no independent and observable definition of the lesion to be detected, the parameter 'sensitivity' is necessarily a model concept (see ref. 7). This introduces a degree of arbitrariness into the simulation context, as effectively as it prevents any absolute measurements in real life, and not surprisingly different investigators tend to produce different results (16). For present purposes the requirement is for a serviceable working value.

The choice of a working value was affected in this case by the need to explain the observed degree of overlap between mammography and palpation in the HIP study, and the observed numbers of women who presented with clinical cancer within a short time of a negative screening examination. The overlap data, from the HIP study, are presented in Table 4. The sensitivity of palpation would be defined correctly in this table as $88/T$ and of mammography as $73/T$, the problem being the unknown value of the grand total (T) and of the numbers of double false negatives in the body of the table.

TABLE 4

Mammography and palpation results in 132 women with lesions subsequently proved to be cancer (HIP)

		Mammogram		
		Positive	*Negative*	*Total*
	Positive	29	59	88
Palpation	*Negative*	44	T–132	T–98
	Total	73	T–73	T

The grand total (T) cannot, of course, be less than 132 (ie $29+59+44$). Simple proportionality in the table, that is assuming that the probability of detection by one test is independent of the probability of detection by the other, would set a grand total at about 222. In general we would expect two tests for the same disease to be positively correlated and would usually expect the total to be substantially greater than that suggested on a null-association hypothesis. However, the total number of cancer cases in the study group among women actually attending for screening was only 223: the extra 91 presenting spontaneously following a previous negative examination. Some of these may genuinely have had no tumour at the time of the examination, which would reduce our expectations for the grand total even further; others, with 'missed' tumours, may yet present themselves later.

We are left in some uncertainty, but the data as a whole suggest that the grand total must be somewhere in the range 200–240. On this basis a (rather optimistic) 45 per cent sensitivity was attributed to palpation and a 40 per cent sensitivity to mammography with respect to pre-clinical cancers, together with higher sensitivities (60 per cent) for any so-far-not-presented clinical cancers. In practice the uncertainty is not critical to the simulation exercise because the natural history of the early stages was subsequently adjusted to the allocated sensitivity values, until the real-life outputs were successfully mimicked.

Specificities for both tests were set at 99·65 per cent; that is, 0·35 per cent of normals would become false positives and have an additional biopsy. This number was set rather arbitrarily following some preliminary arithmetic based on the HIP results, and upon the assumption that perhaps half of the biopsies in the HIP study group were 'additional' if not definitely 'unnecessary'. There are at present no hard data against which to check the 'false-positive' rate except to say that the real value cannot have been greater than twice the value chosen. Fortunately, the specificities of the procedures are sufficiently high, and the number of false positives is sufficiently small, not to interact substantially with other elements of the simulation. The outcomes will thus be sufficient for describing the *relative* medical hazards of alternative regimes, and if further data become available the outcome values can be adjusted simply and linearly without the necessity to re-run the simulation.

(c) Fatalities

As explained earlier it was necessary to readjust initially allocated transfer-rates in order to shorten the process from onset to death. The early stage of follow-up at which significant mortality improvements appeared in the New York experiment, necessitated the premiss that a significant proportion of the cases detected through screening would otherwise have been dead within about four years of entry to the study; this probably means within about two years of detection through screening. Indeed, a problem arose in that these adjustments threatened to produce fatality curves so steep as to be incompatible with those reported in other studies (15, 17, 18, 19, 20) and in the end a compromise was necessary. The terms of this compromise were described earlier; its outcomes, in simulation, were as follows.

First, the effect of simulating four combined examinations (mammography plus palpation) at ages 50–53 in all 10,000 women in the cohort, was a total breast cancer death saving of 24 cases, at age 95. This had earlier reached a peak of 25 cases at age 65, fifteen years after the first screen, and most of the benefit had been attained after ten years of follow-up, when the gap between screened and unscreened was 22. This outcome can be regarded as a reasonably good mimicry of the interim seven-year values recorded in New York, the scaled-down expectation from which was 21 deaths saved at seven years. Details are given in Table 5.

TABLE 5

Numbers of breast cancer deaths saved within successive follow-up periods from entry. Comparison of simulation and observation

	0	1	2	3	4	5	6	7	8 ...	10	... 15 ...	45
						Year of follow-up						
Simulation	0	0	1	2	5	8	11	15	18	22	25	23
New York, reduced*	0	–	–2	+2	7	10	–	21	...	Not yet available ...		

* Scaling down is by factor 0·536 as described in text.

The total of 467 simulated deaths when no screening was performed were divided between high grade and low grade in the ratio 258:209. The deaths saved in the HIP mimicry were almost equally divided between the two classes, suggesting that the screening programme was more effective for preventing deaths from low-grade cancer, than from high-grade cancer, in a ratio of about 1·4:1. No reports of results according to histological gradings have so far been reported from the New York experiment but the simulated result has some parallels with respect to recorded survivals of metastatic and non-metastatic cases and the simulation may be regarded as having at least a qualitative relationship with real-life expectations.

The performance of the simulated procedures in terms of single and double positives and negatives is set out in Table 6. Table 6 does not include a number of cases detected by one or other test after having been missed by both on a previous occasion, or a number of so-far-not-presented clinical cases. Because of these omissions (dictated by limitations to the capacity of the simulation system) the

TABLE 6

Detection of pre-clinical cancers by simulated HIP screening programme

		Mammogram		
		Positive	*Negative*	*Total*
	Positive	14 (16)	27 (33)	41 (49)
Palpation	*Negative*	16 (25)	35	51
	Total	30 (41)	62	92

Scaled-down HIP findings in parenthesis.

comparison in Table 6 with scaled-down HIP results is intended to show compatibility with the observed *relative* distribution, rather than absolute comparability.

In the simulated programme the resource costs were 1,524 examinations per death saved, while in the actual HIP scheme, so far as can be determined from the published results, costs were about 1,695 tests per death saved.

Over-all, the outcomes of this simulation constitute a picture which corresponds reasonably well with data on incidence prevalence and mortality in the general population, with case fatalities of treated clinical cancer, and with the results of applying experimental screening procedures in real life. The terms of the simulation, and the specifications of the natural history and the screening procedures in particular, therefore probably constitute a sufficiently accurate basis from which to explore the likely outcomes of alternative levels of investment and alternative patterns of deployment.

EXTRAPOLATION TO REALISTIC SCREENING PROGRAMMES

(*a*) *Effect of age*

The HIP results suggested that the mortality benefits of screening might be limited to women over 50 years. This might in part have been due to lower yields at the younger ages and so a series of simulation experiments was carried out in which the age of testing was varied. This series was carried out on sets of five tests (as opposed to the four for the primary simulation), applied successively at ages 40–44, 45–49, 50–54, 55–59, and 60–64. The respective numbers of breast cancer deaths saved in the whole cohort were 18, 21, 24, 26, and 26.

This pattern follows closely the prevalence of undetected cancer in the different age-groups and confirms general expectations that relatively late screening will save more lives than screening carried out at earlier ages, although, of course, lives with shorter natural expectations. However, these results do not explain fully the age-dependence of the HIP results. So far as subsequent predictions are concerned these findings suggest that simulated extensions to lower age-groups will tend to exaggerate probable real-life benefits. Furthermore, since it will be shown later that substantial control of breast cancer mortality is dependent upon our ability to extend effective screening across all the age-groups, the numerical uncertainties of the HIP results in the under-50s appear as one of the crucial uncertainties which we shall have to try to answer in the future.

(*b*) *Effects of successive screening procedures*

Curtailment of the HIP simulation to a single examination at age 50, that is omitting the subsequent tests at 51, 52, and 53, saved nine of the twenty-four deaths avoided by the full HIP-simulation set. Thus, the mean marginal benefit of the subsequent tests was only five deaths each, a little more than half the effectiveness of the first test. This is presumably due to an accumulated availability of relatively slow-growing tumours, at the first examination.

The questions arise (i) how this initial pattern of diminishing returns might progress as a series is extended, and (ii) what results might be obtained through varying the intervals between the examinations.

A first set of simulated experiments was carried out using a lengthening series of annual tests (0, 1, 2, 3, 7, 15, 20, 30). The age range was extended in both directions, but more rapidly upwards than downwards. The single-test programme was offered at age 48, the seven-test programme between ages 45 and 51 and the thirty-test programme between ages 41 and 70. At these ages the single-test programme saved 8·3 lives in the full cohort, the second saved an extra 5·0, and the third an extra 4·2. Thereafter the curve of incremental benefits flattened out and between seven and fifteen tests the mean incremental benefit was 4·1. Beyond this there was a secondary fall to 3·6 in the 15–20 range and to 3·2 in the 20–30 range. The secondary decline in marginal benefits is probably due to extensions into younger age-groups where the prevalence is low, and into older age-groups where deaths from other causes, even in cancer patients, are increasingly likely. The age-specific inaccuracies of the simulation, compared with HIP, would suggest that the secondary fall might be somewhat greater in real life than this set of simulation experiments indicates.

The first examination was also the cheapest in terms of the number of tests per life saved, namely 1,124 tests. The marginal cost associated with the second test was 1,856 tests per life saved; thereafter the cost remained fairly constant between 2,050 and 2,200 tests per life saved. Hazards to the patient rose in a similar pattern; a first test resulted in 7·8 additional non-cancer biopsies per life saved, a second test 12·8, and subsequent tests between 14·3 and 15·5.

The total cost of a seven-test series was 1,847 tests and 12·9 extra biopsies per life saved resulting in a 7·4 per cent saving of total mortality. A fifteen-test series cost 1,950 tests and 13·6 biopsies per life with a total saving of 14·4 per cent of mortality. A thirty-test series cost 2,022 tests and 14·1 biopsies per life with a total saving of 25·0 per cent.

It should be remarked that the 25 per cent saving of mortality associated with a thirty-test sequence refers only to the contingency of 100 per cent attendance. The New York experiment suggests that it may in fact be difficult to obtain more than 50 per cent continuing attendance. The simulation therefore suggests that even with massive investment, simple extension of the HIP technique cannot be expected to reduce mortality from breast cancer by more than about 12 per cent.

This relatively unfavourable forecast is supported by the finding that in the thirty-test simulation 83 per cent of all cancers were in fact detected by a screening test, suggesting that at this level of investment the main constraint is probably set by the properties of the disease rather than the efficiency of the screening examination.

A second series of simulated experiments was carried out in which a four-test series was deployed first at single-year intervals, then at two-year intervals, three-year intervals, and so on up to ten-year intervals. The experiment was related to the question of the optimal deployment of a limited resource and the question whether the disproportionate success of a first examination could be repeated in subsequent examinations provided they were not too close to each other.

The single-year spacing (ages 54–57) saved 24·6 deaths from a total of 467 in the absence of screening. Spacings of two, three, four, five, and six years saved 29·5, 32·9, 34·6, and 35·4 lives. Single-year spacings cost 1,425 examinations per life saved while two-year, three-year, and four-year spacings cost 1,183, 1,056, and 996 respectively. Beyond this point the costs were all between 955 and 970 tests per life saved.

(c) Marginal benefits of mammography

A serious attempt to lower the mortality from breast cancer in England and Wales through a simple extension of the HIP scheme would require a large investment. For example, a 50 per cent take-up of an offer of thirty annual examinations might reduce mortality by 12 per cent and would require the provision of about $4\cdot4\times10^6$ examinations each year. (There are $8\cdot8\times10^6$ women aged 40–69 years in England and Wales.)

A single-stream specialized clinic can provide fewer than twenty combined palpation and mammographic examinations per half-day session and allowing for inefficiencies of usage such a programme would require about 600 such streams.

Very approximately, the equipment for each stream would cost £10,000, premises or their adaptation another £10,000, while salaries (two regular non-medical staff, plus locums, plus consultant cover, plus secretarial support) together with consumables and publicity might amount to £10,000 per annum. The provision of £12 million for capital investment over the course of a few years and annual running costs rising rapidly towards £6 million per annum, may not be easy to find, not to mention the problems of providing for the training of 1,200–1,500 necessary additional staff. Furthermore, a scheme of this extent can scarcely be envisaged until the radiation dose exposure has been consistently reduced to not more than 1 rad per examination: perhaps with an increase in costs.

In all these respects the main constraints upon the growth of the service are associated with mammography rather than palpation. We therefore need to inquire into the extent of the marginal benefits of mammography over palpation alone in the context of an extended scheme. Many permutations of this theme could be examined but in the first instance a series of simulation experiments was carried out into the effects of omitting mammography altogether and comparing the results with those of the combined tests.

First it was found that repetition of the simulated HIP study (four-tests), but with the mammograms omitted saved 70 per cent of the death-savings of the full regime. This corresponds well with the relative detection performance of palpation alone, compared with palpation plus mammography, in the actual study. However, it was found in the New York study that cases detected by mammogram had a better subsequent prognosis than cases detected by palpation. It could be argued (although it does not *necessarily* follow) that the cases detected by mammogram are those among whom the chief benefit of early detection is concentrated.

This consideration could certainly affect the interpretation of the simulations which follow and the question of differential benefit according to mode of detection is therefore an important research issue for purposes of planning in the future. However, if for the time being we do not differentiate prognostically between palpation detected and mammography-detected cases, the indications are as follows.

First, the *proportional* marginal benefit of mammography plus palpation, over palpation alone, fell as the series of examinations was extended. For a single examination, 39·7 per cent of the savings were lost if mammography was omitted and in three, seven, fifteen, and thirty-test extensions the losses were 34·2, 31·3, 27·2, and 21·2 per cent. Replacement of the mammograms recovered the savings at a cost which arose from 2,826 mammograms per death saved for a single examination regime, rising steadily through 7,161 for the fifteen-test series to 9,602 for the thirty-test series. Each of these values refers to the full series as specified; that is the costs are marginal only in the sense of providing mammography over and above palpation and not in the sense of providing a longer test-series over and above a shorter one. When marginal costing techniques are computed in the two dimensions simultaneously, mammography appears in an even less favourable light. For example, a simulated comparison was made between the provision of thirty double exami-nations and a regime consisting of thirty palpations but only fifteen mammograms. At this ultimate extension each additional death saved would cost 10,267 mammograms. Radiation exposure on this scale and at recently prevalent doses, would almost certainly cause more cancers than were cured as a result of detection.

All these figures must be treated with the quantitative reservations indicated earlier, but in qualitative terms they probably supply a fair assessment of the pattern of changes in the marginal benefit of mammography as a service is extended. It appears quite unlikely that present mammographic techniques can supply the basis for a substantial control of breast cancer mortality, and the diminishing marginal benefits of two tests over one as a service is extended will probably enforce an increasing reliance on palpation techniques.

THE EFFECTS OF PRE-SCREENING

Another approach to a discrepancy between resource requirements and availability is to limit applications selectively to those groups most likely to benefit. These groups may possibly, although not necessarily, be identified as those with the highest initial risks.

To some extent the high-risk woman can be identified on social/ biological criteria related to previous reproductive and menstrual histories but a single estimation of urinary aetiocholanolone levels appears also to differentiate between high-risk and low-risk women. The problem with this test, as indicated earlier, is that it also possibly selects women with relatively high-grade tumours and relatively poor prognosis. Certainly it has this implication once a tumour has been found. In previous runs of the simulation system it was confirmed that the natural history generated equal numbers of high-grade and low-grade tumours and more deaths among high-grade tumours than among low-grade ones, as indeed it was designed to do, but that screening was more effective among the low-grade than among the high-grade cancers. The ratio between the percentage saved of low-grade cancer deaths and the percentage saved of high-grade cancer deaths was 1·7:1 for a single examination (palpation + mammography). On further investigation it was found that the relative effectiveness of screening in low-grade and high-grade tumours, changed as the investment was increased and as the screening programme was extended, and when a series of twenty annual tests was performed, the above ratio had fallen to 1·2:1. The pattern is therefore complex, presumably because the potential benefits to the low-grade tumours are exhausted relatively early, while the limits for high-grade tumours are not reached until later.

If aetiocholanolone levels do in fact tend to select high-grade tumours, their disadvantage in this respect would probably diminish as the investment increased.

Much will depend of course upon the selectivity of the pre-screening test, or combinations of tests, which it is proposed to use. It is scarcely possible to obtain quantitative values at the present time, especially those which could be applied separately to high-grade and low-grade tumours. Therefore, a simulation study can, for the time being, supply only a crude qualitative prediction of the likely outcomes.

For purposes of such an inquiry it was postulated that a reasonable medium-term expectation of the urinary steroid test might be to select one-third of the population in whom one-half of the breast tumours would occur. The simulated screening test was therefore allocated a 33 per cent sensitivity and the high-risk group was given twice the onset rate of the remaining low-risk group. It was further supposed that the ratio of low-grade to high-grade onsets would be distributed unequally between the two groups; these requirements were met by allocating the basic onset rate for low-grade tumours equally to high-risk and low-risk women, while the transfer rates for high-grade tumours were set at double the basic rate in the high-risk women and half the basic rate in the low-risk group. This combination of ratios retained the same net over-all transfer rates for the whole cohort whether or not the pre-screening test was actually applied.

Comparable screening programmes of 1, 5, 10, 20, and 30 combined examinations (palpation plus mammography) were carried out in low-risk and high-risk normals, and the results compared in each case with the results of no screening procedure at all. When the above successive regimes were limited to the high-risk group, the successive percentage savings of total mortality in high- and low-risk groups together were 1·2, 3·0, 5·2, 9·1, and 12·4. When screening was limited to the low-risk group of women the savings were almost identical at 1·2, 3·2, 5·4, 9·4, and 12·8 per cent, although at the cost of screening twice as many women. The marginal costs, in terms of extra examinations carried out per extra death saved were 617, 1,230, 1,327, 1,398, and 1,493 in successive extensions in the high-risk group. For the low-risk group, the values were 1,114, 2,452, 2,712, 2,861, and 3,101.

This confirms the complexity of the pattern referred to earlier, but it is clear that, despite the potential disadvantage of the pre-screening technique in selecting the more malignant tumours, surveillance of high-risk women gives much better returns for investment at every level. It is noteworthy, in particular, that the advantage increases as the service extends. Selective screening is thus not to be seen only as a measure to be applied in an interim period of deficient resources; its advantages increase as investment increases. Indeed, once the total population has received a limited number of examinations, say four or five, *all* resources subsequently made available are most profitably expended on the high-risk group. If pre-screening is developed to a more selective level than that used in the simulation, this conclusion must apply with even greater force.

SELECTIVE REGIMES

It would be fruitless on present evidence to try to optimize formally a selective allocation of resources at different levels of investment, but the simulations carried out so far indicate the principles on which this might be done. Thus, there are grounds (in the context of limited resources) for spacing examinations at intervals of up to about four years, for detecting and concentrating resources upon high-risk groups, and for extending palpation regimes at the expense of mammography. A simulation exercise was carried out in which (i) a single pre-screening examination was carried out; (ii) surveillance of the low-risk group was carried out at four-year intervals between 42 and 70 years, eight tests in all, and (iii) screening of the high-risk group was carried out at two-year intervals over the same age period, sixteen tests in all, and (iv) for both groups palpation was carried out at each examination, but mammography only on alternate occasions.

The end result was a 17·6 per cent saving of all deaths, a substantial fraction of the 25 per cent saving achieved for a far larger investment (see earlier) of thirty double examinations in all groups. The cost per life saved under this selective regime amounted to 117 urine tests, 1,068 palpations, and 542 mammograms.

If 50 per cent of the adult female population of England and Wales could be induced to undertake such a regime, the saving of 8·8 per cent of current mortality would amount to 1,040 deaths saved each year, at an annual cost of 120,000 urine tests, 1·1 million palpations, and 0·6 million mammograms. In practice, there would be a wide distribution of attendance patterns between full attendance and no attendance at all, and because of the way in which diminishing returns are distributed we might expect a better result from this than from the 'two-population' model. Consequently a second simulation was carried out in which, as before, all women were subjected to pre-screening, but in which the subsequent attendance pattern was set at 50 per cent on each separate occasion. Each attendance in each woman was thus regarded as independent of the previous and following attendances. This model is, of course, as artificial as the previous one, but gives some indication of the maximum additional savings which might be obtained. These amounted to 13·0 per cent of total mortality instead of 8·8 per cent. If we set our real-life expectations at a point midway between the results of the 'two-population' model and the second 'Poissonian' model we might anticipate a saving of about 11 per cent of mortality. Having regard to the results of previous simulations, and the complexity of the approach which was necessary in order to attain this 11 per cent we should anticipate that any investment beyond that computed for the selective programme would encounter rapidly diminishing returns and steeply rising marginal costs. Consequently, a target of 11 per cent saving of current mortality is probably the most that we could reasonably set ourselves within current and foreseeable limits of technique, staff, and finance.

Discussion

The process of converting a technical procedure to a definitive service is a complex process. In the first place it involves a translation of individual patient-care objectives (doing one's best for each patient in the light of present knowledge and resources), to population-based objectives (reducing the mortality rate), and basing judgements upon the feasibility of meeting them. In the second place it requires a relatively exact quantitative consideration of a wide range of elements which at the individual level are expressed in qualitative terms, namely errors, prognoses, the effectiveness of treatment, attendance and default rates, the risks and consequences of unnecessary treatment and investigation, natural expectations of life, costs savings, manpower, skills, and so on. Complex combinations of the constraints upon prospective success must be taken into account.

These approaches are sometimes characterized as 'cost-effectiveness' or 'cost-benefit' studies, the first when the problem is defined as that of finding the cheapest way of achieving a predefined effect, and the second when a degree of planning freedom is allowed to the level and quality of the benefit. The notion of a cost/benefit *ratio* is also sometimes invoked. However, it can be misleading to use an arithmetic term here since it is sometimes taken to mean that we must reduce everything to commensurable and divisible (for example cash) terms. In many situations it is better to assemble a planning proposal on the basis of two separate balance sheets. The first should set out the observed or predicted health results as a numerical statement of qualitatively defined benefits and harmful effects; the second should set out the cash costs and the discounted cash savings within one or more appropriate budgetary frames of reference.

It is usually unnecessary, often impossible, and sometimes harmful to try to set out the whole relationship in cash terms alone. Health-care benefits can be considered economically as 'goods' in their own right, and their economic justification should not always have to be stated in cash or similar (for example, working days, anticipated tax payment, productivity) terms.

This, at any rate, is the view which has guided the approach presented here, to the extent that very little attempt has been made to attach cash costs even to resource requirements. Indeed, at certain levels of proposed investment, absolute availability constraints (for example, manpower) make this quite unnecessary for purposes of reaching conclusions. This is not to say that when the limits of desirable and feasible policies have been drawn, cash studies have no place. Clearly they have. However, the (cash-) economic considerations can enter only at a secondary level, *after* the nature of the medical-care 'goods' has been thoroughly assessed and this is the purpose of the study reported here.

The conclusions drawn, by the very nature of the process used, have the characteristics of predictions and recommendations rather than facts. Facts were the starting point. The conclusions come under three main headings relating to (i) the probable effects of initial and extended investments in breast cancer screening programmes in Britain or in similar countries; (ii) the constraints which would be encountered, and the changed deployment of resource which would necessarily occur as a service developed; and (iii) the needs for particular items of information which would emerge during development, and the research investment which would be required in order to meet them.

(i) The probable effects of a straightforward extension of a programme of mammography and palpation can be described briefly as disappointing. Maximum mortality control, assuming an optimistic 50 per cent uptake of a screening offer and based on the probably unrealistic assumption of thirty successive annual examinations, could be expected to be about 12 per cent. Within the next ten to fifteen years nothing approaching this saving could be envisaged and there is virtually no hope of achieving a substantial effect upon mortality in the short or medium term. The cash and resource costs of an extended programme appear to be large. Dowdy, Barker, Legasse, Sperling, Zeldis, and Longmire (21) suggested that in the USA, with an over-40 female population of 38×10^6, a programme of this extent could cost about \$622 million, annually.

Scaling down according to population, exchange rate, and a 50 per cent assumed uptake translates this to £36 million annually in England and Wales. The rough estimates presented earlier in this paper suggested that NHS prices would be much less than this, probably not more than £10–12 million per annum. On this basis lives might be saved at a cost of about £8,000 each. A selective programme, aiming at a 10 per cent reduction in mortality, might achieve this at £2,000–3,000 per life. This is much less than Dowdy *et al.*'s estimate suggests: about £27,000 per life saved in a large-scale, non-selective, specialist-manned, American-priced context. Kodlin (22) has also produced cost estimates in the American scene. His projections are very much less than those of Dowdy *et al.*, £700–2,000 per life saved. However, this is in the context of a very limited programme, corresponding in size with the HIP experiment, and seems to depend upon unrealistic assumptions, including an extremely optimistic estimate of sensitivity (95 per cent).

An extended thirty-test programme in England and Wales, which might prevent approximately 1,300 breast cancer deaths (out of 11,000) would need also to be set against about 13,000 additional biopsies and an indeterminate number of induced cancers. The cancer-induction problem will be considered in more detail later, but the biopsies alone would mean that approximately 5 per cent of all women, or about 10 per cent of participants, would eventually acquire an additional and probably unnecessary surgical procedure.

There are of course other considerations than those treated in the simulation and some of them tend to place screening in a more favourable light. First it can be argued that mortality savings are not to be seen as the sole criterion and that it is possible to provide short but useful prolongations of life without affecting grossly the cumulative death statistics. The quality of life may be influenced favourably, there may be psychological advantages to an aggressive approach to the disease, the secondary benefits of health education are a worthwhile bonus, and the provision of a service may be a necessary preliminary to fruitful research. Each is accepted as valid and it is certainly not implied in the present analysis that mortality statistics are to be regarded as a sole criterion. It is held, however, that they are an important criterion of success and in this disease can certainly be regarded as a valid index if not a comprehensive evaluation, of the performance of a service.

The question of unnecessary biopsy also raises a subtle question. This is because the notion of an unnecessary biopsy for a suspect lump in the breast is difficult to appreciate against a background of clinical practice and in the light of the basic surgical aphorism that 'no lady should have a lump'. It is conceded of course that excision represents good clinical practice for lumps which present spontaneously and it may seem unrealistic to suggest that the rules should be different for lumps which are discovered by invitation. Moreover some lumps, even when not cancers, are presumably best removed. Nevertheless, although it is seldom possible in an individual case to say that removal was unnecessary, we have no option, from a planning point of view, but to regard additional removals of non-symptomatic lumps which would otherwise not have presented, as a net cost to be set against the benefits.

A similar set of considerations arises in relation to radiation exposure, where it may be difficult at first to accept that a procedure which delivers a dose commensurate with that delivered in many routine clinical investigations has in this case to be treated differently. It may be validly argued, moreover, that estimates of the radiation hazard are subject to gross uncertainties, being based largely upon extrapolations from a variety of dissimilar exposure experiences and a pervading assumption of a linear relationship between the total dose delivered and the cancers caused, whatever the distribution of the radiation in terms of people, the numbers of doses, the intensity and quality of radiation, and the intervals between doses. The latent interval of the postulated effect is also uncertain and most of our data relate to whole body radiation.

However, there are two sources of information which are relevant to mammography in a reasonably direct manner. First, McKenzie (1965) discovered 13 cases of breast cancer within ten years of pneumothorax treatment for pulmonary tuberculosis in 271 women, compared with one among 510 women with (presumably) comparable risk but without pneumothorax treatment or repeated fluoroscopy. Doses were probably around 2,000 r per woman, in total, and the dose/response ratio was approximately 25 breast cancers per million per rad. Wanebo, Johnson, Sato, and Thorslund (24) studied breast cancer occurrences within twenty years of single dose exposures in Hiroshima and Nagasaki. Breast cancer has a low natural incidence in Japan but the dose-response curve suggests an effect, within twenty years, of about 30 cases per million per rad. The doses which these affected Japanese women received were mainly in the range 10–200 r. Thus, while the question of linearity remains unsettled the best evidence we have suggests a total induction rate in the region of 30 cases per million per rad within twenty years of exposure, or between one-tenth and one-eighth of the effect of equivalent whole body radiation. On this basis a delivery of $4\cdot4\times10^6$ examinations per annum (required for a 50 per cent uptake of a thirty-examination offer, at 5 r per examination), might generate up to 660 cancers. Some of the affected women would die before the tumour actually appeared but the prospect is nevertheless daunting. There is little doubt that a large reduction in dosage in all units to levels at least as low as those presently achieved in the best (eg 0·5 r) would be mandatory before a general scheme on this scale could be launched.

(ii) The chief constraints upon providing an extended screening programme, whether in terms of capital costs, materials, salaries, premises, clinical throughputs, or hazards, are associated with mammography. Furthermore, the ratio between the marginal gains of mammography and its marginal costs and hazards, will decrease as the service extends. Important questions remain about mortality savings in mammography-detected cases compared with palpation-detected cases, but if palpation has any value at all the relative place of mammography will decline as a service grows. If a service is in fact developed and extended, and meets familiar pressures of a growing demand in the face of limited resources, it will be forced into an increasing reliance upon palpation methods and a limited and selective usage of mammograms. The results of the HIP experiment may not have been too useful here. Instead, we would need to measure quite accurately the effectiveness, hazards, and costs of an extended palpation programme using staff other than doctors, and of teaching self-palpation, together with the marginal benefits, risks, and costs of a selective and limited use of mammography, superimposed upon this background.

We can anticipate in addition that more and more reliance will be placed upon selectively prescribed programmes of surveillance, and that initially over-ambitious targets will be replaced eventually by the hopes of saving about 10 per cent of current deaths.

Finally, if after a period of twenty-five years of development, no new diagnostic or treatment techniques had appeared we should anticipate a demand for a reappraisal. In the light of the large annual expenditure incurred by this time and the limited (and perhaps non-demonstrable) benefits, it will probably be decided to redirect a substantial part of the investment into basic research.

(iii) It is easy to suggest that if the main effect of such a large expenditure would be the eventual diversion of commensurate resources into basic research, we should do so now without the preliminary expense. Certainly we should recognize that any hopes of substantial control through screening will depend upon far more accurate and economic screening and pre-screening procedures than we have at present, probably combined with more effective treatment for early lesions, and any reasonable research proposals in this area, as well as those concerned with primary causation and prevention, deserve very high priority.

However, obtaining timely research results in a specific area cannot depend only upon a policy of supplying resources in response to research proposals. In this field in particular, where present evidence does not justify the establishment of a definitive service, but where the scientific and operational issues can scarcely be approached in the absence of a service of some kind, this is a special and urgent organizational problem. The situation must be met through the establishment of a mechanism for running a large-scale, although localized, experimental service. That is to say, the service must be established under, and remain under, scientific direction in a manner which permits the incorporation and control of a continuing series of inquiries and experiments: for example into the effectiveness of different pre-selection techniques or into the relative benefits of different regimes of recall and review. A need for a 'planning and control agency' of this kind is asserted simply because there is no other physical solution. It must consist of committed and probably whole-time workers (although they may undertake related responsibilities in addition) and they must have adequate powers covering the deployment of a budget and the negotiation and supervision of a co-ordinated plan. This work *cannot* be done by a committee nor by a group limited to an advisory function. If its exact position and powers are difficult to envisage within the present administration of the health service, then that is a defect of the system, and a means of adapting the system to the need will have been found.

Summary

The planning of a breast cancer screening service is affected by two sets of problems, namely: (i) a series of quantitative uncertainties about the error rates of the two main screening procedures, their acceptability to the population at risk, the extent of the radiation hazard, the effectiveness of early treatment in the several varieties of disease, and the selectivity of pre-screening procedures; and (ii) the problem of extrapolation from the (experimental) circumstances in which we have some direct knowledge about the important matters, to the context of a full-scale service, with various administrative options relating to the total investment, the age at deployment, and the intervals between tests. This study is an exploration, using computer simulation, of the interactions between the options and the uncertainties.

The first stage of the process was a repeated adjustment of the input parameters until the outputs matched available data. The available data included age-specific registration and death rates, case fatality rates according to grade and stage, and the results of the New York (HIP) controlled experiment on the effects of palpation and mammography. The inputs specified the natural history of the disease, the effectiveness of the treatment and the sensitivity of the screening tests.

Extrapolation of the simulation to conditions envisaged in an extended breast screening service indicated the following: (i) A straightforward extension of the HIP pattern of screening will encounter diminishing returns and a fall in the marginal value of additional tests. (ii) This fall will be encountered in two stages, an earlier one over the range of the first four or five tests, and a later one at extensions beyond about twenty tests per woman per lifetime. (iii) The marginal value of added mammography over palpation alone will fall as the service is extended and will reach a point where additional mammograms may be doing more harm than good. (iv) Pre-selection techniques, even when not very selective, can greatly increase the economy of a screening scheme despite a possible tendency to select women with less tractable tumours. (v) The value of pre-selection techniques tends to increase as the service extends; they are not to be seen simply as a stop-gap during an initial period of limited resources. (vi) Having regard to the limited acceptability of screening procedures, their high costs, the pattern of diminishing returns, and the hazards of radiation and of unnecessary biopsy, a reasonable service target (within present technology) may be a reduction of breast cancer mortality by about one-tenth. (vii) The main questions to which developmental research should be directed, if a service is in fact to be developed, relate to a clarification of the marginal value of a limited mammographic regime superimposed upon a more intensive palpation regime, the effectiveness of health education and of self-palpation, the selectivity/sensitivity of pre-screening tests and the effectiveness of early treatment in women under 45.

References

1. HARRIS, D. L., GREENING, W. P., and AICHROTH, P. M. (1966). 'Infra-red in the diagnosis of a lump in the breast', *Br. J. Cancer*, **20**, 710–21.

2. JONES, C. H. (1969). 'Interpretation problems in thermography of the female breast' in *Medical Thermography; Proc. of Boerhaven Course for Post-graduate Medical Education* (Leiden, 1968). *Bibl. Radiol.*, no. 5, 96–108 (Basel, New York: Karger).

3. —— and DRAPER, J. W. (1970). 'A comparison of infra-red photography and thermography in the detection of mammary carcinoma', *Br. J. Radiol.* **43**, 507–16.

4. SHAPIRO, S., STRAX, P., VENET, L., and VENET, W. (1973). 'Changes in 5-year breast cancer mortality in a breast cancer screening programme', *Seventh National Cancer Conference Proceedings*, pp. 663–78 (Philadelphia, London: Lippincott).

5. BEIR (National Research Council Advisory Committee on the Biological Effects of Ionizing Radiations) (1972). *The Effect on Populations of Exposure to Low-Levels of Ionizing Radiation* (particular reference made to footnote (*b*), table 3–2 on p. 171) (Washington: National Academy of Sciences, National Research Council).

6. SHAPIRO, S. (1975). *Bull. N.Y. Acad. Med.* **51**, in press (and personal communication).

7. KNOX, E. G. (1973). 'A simulation system for screening procedures', in McLachlan, G. (ed.), *The Future—and Present Indicatives, Problems and Progress in Medical Care*, Ninth Series (Oxford University Press for the Nuffield Provincial Hospitals Trust).

8. DOLL, R., MUIR, C. S., and WATERHOUSE, J. A. H. (1970). *Cancer Incidence in Five Continents* (Berlin, Heidelberg, New York: International Union against Cancer; Springer-Verlag).

9. CHIEF MEDICAL OFFICER OF ENGLAND AND WALES (1966). *Annual Report* (London: HMSO).

10. REGISTRAR GENERAL OF ENGLAND AND WALES. *Supplement on Cancer 1966–67* (London: HMSO).

11. —— (1971). *Statistical Review* (London: HMSO).

12. BLOOM, H. J. G., RICHARDSON, W. W., and FIELD, J. R. (1970). 'Host resistance and survival in carcinoma of the breast: a study of 104 cases of medullary carcinoma in a series of 1411 cases of breast cancer followed for 20 years', *Br. med. J.* **3,** 181–8.

13. HARTVEIT, F. (1971). 'Prognostic typing in breast cancer', ibid. **4,** 253–7.

14. BLOOM, H. J. G., and FIELD, J. R. (1971). 'Impact of tumour grade and host resistance on survival of women with breast cancer', *Cancer*, **28,** 1580–9.

15. —— (1965). 'The influence of delay on the natural history and prognosis of breast cancer', *Br. J. Cancer*, **19,** 228–62.

16. FURNIVAL, I. G., STEWART, H. J., WEDDELL, J. M., DOVEY, P., GRAVELLE, I. H., EVANS, K. T., and FORREST, A. P. M. (1970). 'Accuracy of screening methods for the diagnosis of breast diseases', *Br. med. J.* **4,** 461–3.

17. BLOOM, H. J. G. (1968). 'Survival of women with untreated breast cancer—past and present', in Forest, A. P. M., and Kunkler, P. B. (eds), *Prognostic Factors in Breast Cancer*.

18. BOND, W. H. (1967). 'The influence of various treatments on survival rates in cancer of the breast', in Jowett, A. S. (ed.), *The Treatment of Carcinoma of the Breast* (Excerpta Medica Foundation).

19. WATERHOUSE, J. A. H. (1974). *Cancer: Handbook of Epidemiology and Prognosis* (Edinburgh: Churchill–Livingstone).

20. BRUCE, J. (1971). 'Operable cancer of the breast. A controlled clinical trial', *Cancer*, **28,** 1443–52.

21. DOWDY, A. H., BARKER, W. F., LAGASSE, L. D., SPERLING, L., ZELDIS, L. J., and LONGMIRE, W. P. (1971). 'Mammography as a screening method for the examination of large populations', ibid. **28,** 1558–62.

22. KODLIN, D. (1972). 'A note on the cost benefit problem in screening for breast cancer', *Meth. Inf. Med.* **11,** 242–7.

23. MACKENZIE, I. (1965). 'Breast cancer following multiple fluoroscopies', *Br. J. Cancer*, **19,** 1–8.

24. WANEBO, C. K., JOHNSON, K. J., SATO, K., and THORSLUND, T. W. (1968). 'Breast cancer after exposure to the atomic bombings of Hiroshima and Nagasaki', *New Engl. J. Med.* **279,** 667–71.

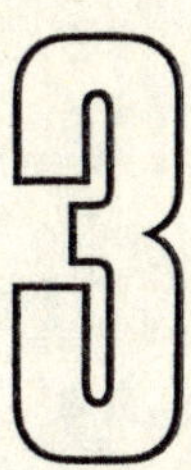

L. J. Opit
BSc, FRCS
Health Services Research Centre
Department of Social Medicine
University of Birmingham

J. Selwyn Crawford
FFARCS
Consultant Anaesthetist
Birmingham Maternity Hospital

Obstetric anaesthesia :
A regional audit

Obstetric anaesthesia :
A regional audit

Introduction

For some years the DHSS has published a triennial report on maternal deaths in England and Wales. This report has been both anecdotal and analytic in nature and has provided information on the numbers and characters of patients dying during childbirth or abortion. The reports have stressed factors which the review committee considered preventable and thus has attempted to guide professional practice.

Although during the last twenty years there has been a steady decline in total mortality, the deaths associated with obstetric anaesthesia have risen both absolutely and relatively. The majority of these deaths are associated with the aspiration of gastric juice and the development of Mendelson's Syndrome (6). Since this cause of death should be largely preventable the observations of the Committee on Maternal Mortality have been a source of some concern to anaesthetists (2). In 1968 the Obstetric Anaesthetists Association was formed and one of its first tasks was to commission an inquiry into the anaesthetist staffing of maternity units. This inquiry was a postal survey carried out by Dr J. Taylor (5) and it revealed a very heavy dependance on junior anaesthetists in many regional obstetric units. It was felt that a more detailed study of the operational features of obstetric anaesthesia including its relationship to serious anaesthetic morbidity was required and the study reported here is the outcome of the concern created by Taylor's earlier inquiry. Since childbirth is common, and anaesthetic death associated with it still quite rare, it was felt that a regional study over a six-month period including every hospital providing maternity services was required to obtain the necessary data and insight. The Birmingham Region was chosen for study because of its size and the availability of interested persons although in many respects it is amongst the better regions in terms of maternal mortality. It was felt that deficiencies in staff or practice revealed, could be assumed to be as bad, possibly worse, elsewhere in the country.

The object of the survey was then to provide detailed factual information from each maternity unit in the Birmingham Region about: (i) The operational characteristics of the obstetric anaesthetic workload, particularly in relation to the availability of staff, time and notice of services, type of assistance available, and obstetric complexity. (ii) Standards of pre-anaesthetic preparation and care. (iii) Anaesthetic techniques. (iv) Technical difficulties and serious early anaesthetic morbidity affecting the mother.

Such a detailed study is very inclined to produce more questions than answers and data available in this paper represent only a part of the completed study which is being published elsewhere (3, 4). Some results of the study are presented here to indicate the potential uses of detailed specialized field studies in arriving at assessments of the quality and quantity of medical services. We were particularly concerned with effecting change in a neglected service and the results are presented towards this end.

METHOD

Data relating to individual items of anaesthetic service were obtained by questionnaire. For each act of anaesthetic service in the obstetric units one questionnaire was completed by the anaesthetist.

The following categories of service were differentiated:

(i) Standby. This item is used to identify the situation where an anaesthetist was called to assist or to await delivery but where no anaesthetic, general or regional, was given by the anaesthetist.

(ii) Regional. This includes both analgesia and anaesthesia by regional block. Only cases where these procedures were carried out by anaesthetic staff were recorded.

(iii) General anaesthesia. Only cases of pregnancy beyond 28 weeks were included and re-admissions with late surgical or gynaecological complications were not recorded. All post-partum sterilizations which occurred while the patients were in the obstetric units were counted but the questionnaire was not completed for these anaesthetics.

THE QUESTIONNAIRE

The questionnaire had been printed by a commercial printer and contained fifty questions. The answer set for each question was provided and the appropriate answer signified mainly by marking a numbered box. Although the questionnaire was long and appeared complex, a preliminary trial at the teaching hospital unit showed that it was possible to complete this document in three to five minutes. Each questionnaire was numbered and the patient's name was not required. Forms were delivered, with a container, before the trial began to all forty-nine hospitals within the Region in which obstetric care was offered. During the period of the trial, 14 July 1972 to 14 January 1973, these forms were collected at regular intervals by specially appointed data supervisors and were replaced by new ones if necessary. The data supervisors, who were qualified midwives, checked the questionnaire to ensure that all appropriate questions had been answered; in addition they examined birth registers or anaesthetic books to discover missing records or unrecorded services. A count of post-partum sterilizations was also made at this time and details entered into a work sheet. Whenever possible details of un-recorded services were obtained from anaesthetists by asking them to complete a questionnaire subsequent to the procedure. Additional data relating to hospital staffing, staff rosters, and equipment were also collected during these visits. During the survey period one of the authors (L. J. O.) personally visited the majority of the units and much additional informal data was obtained.

Each form was checked on arrival at the Health Services Research Centre and data transferred from the questionnaire on to IBM 80-column cards. Each individual anaesthetic service contact required two such cards. All forms were filed numerically within group order for ease of subsequent search.

The IBM cards were verified and written to a magnetic tape file. Data analysis was conducted on this file by an IBM computer using programs written in Autocode or Fortran.

Results

AVAILABLE RESOURCES

Before considering data related to the use of anaesthetic services in obstetrics, it is necessary to look briefly at the nature and distribution of the beds used for obstetrics in the Region under study for it is quite obvious that the organization of the obstetric beds and the availability of anaesthetists will help to determine the evolution of the clinical practice of both obstetrics and obstetric anaesthesia. Thus

where a large portion of obstetric beds in an administrative group are
in GP hospitals, the case-load in the consultant unit might tend to
contain a concentration of the more difficult obstetric problems so
that in looking at anaesthetic workload rates it is necessary to
express these service rates as function of all births in the group.

We have identified two types of units and three classes of beds.
Firstly, cottage hospitals staffed by GPs, usually quite small hospitals
and with no resident anaesthetic or obstetric staff. Secondly there are
units situated in a district hospital setting; these will have consultant
obstetric staff in charge and resident staff in obstetrics probably
available as well. The anaesthetic staff however is usually shared with
other surgical units although in a few cases, in large units they are
attached on a specific work rota. These consultant units may also
have a GP obstetric unit associated with them.

Data relating to these observations are set out in Table 1. There are
eighteen groups, one of them associated with the teaching hospital.
Where a group contains two or more separate consultant units these
are shown separately so that the staffing position can be displayed for
each unit. The table also contains the number of specifically allocated
sessions for consultant anaesthetists per week at the time of the study
and the grade of the anaesthetic staff on emergency roster for the
consultant units. The groups have been arranged in descending order
of size as determined by the total number of obstetric beds. The distribution of beds is seen to be extraordinarily variable. In eight
groups 30 per cent or more of the beds are situated in cottage
hospitals while in four groups less than half of the obstetric beds are
under the control of consultant obstetric staff. On the other hand
three groups have no general practitioner allocated obstetric beds and
one of these groups is in a rural setting.

The table also supports the earlier study of Taylor (5) in showing a
heavy reliance on junior staff grades for first emergency cover and
the significance of this will be examined later. Apart from the teaching group only three groups had senior staff regularly available on
emergency first call, and apart from the teaching group, only four
groups had three or more sessions allocated specifically to consultant
anaesthetists. The grade of facilities shown in the table refers to the
labour wards and operating theatres and represents a purely sub-
jective assessment by the authors of this paper and the data supervisors.

This evaluation can be supported in some degree by noting that

TABLE 1

Distribution of beds and staff by administrative groups

Group	Total beds	Bed distribution (%) Cottage hospital	GP unit	Consultant unit	Emergency roster 1st call	2nd call	Allocated consultant sessions (weekly)	Grade of facilities
A	241	0	22	78	SHO/R/SR	SHO/R/SR	2 (epid. only)	L
					R	CA	2	A
					R	C	–	BA
B	218	18	11	71	SHO/R	R	2	A
C	195	0	7	93	R	C	–	BA
					SHO/R	C	3	L
D	182	30	12	58	R/SR	C	9	A
E	181	0	0	100	SHO/R	SHO	2	BA
					SHO	SHO	–	BA
F	167	13	17	70	R	SHO	1	L
G	128	37	18	45	R/SHO	C	6	A/L
H	115	49	19	32	R	C	1	A
I	105	42	0	58	SHO/R	C	0	A/BA
J	101	0	0	100	SHO/R	SR/C	0	BA
K	94	35	0	65	R	C	2	CR
L	91	43	19	38	SHO/CA/R	C	0	BA
M	82	27	0	73	R	C	3	A
N	73	52	0	48	SHO/R	C	0	A
O	72	30	0	70	R	C	1	BA/A
P	64	0	20	80	SHO/R	C	1	CR
Q	48	0	0	100	SHO/R	C	0	A
Teaching group	170	0	20	80	R/SR	C	11	L

Key
C = Consultant   SHO = Senior house officer   L = Luxurious
CA = Clinical assistant   R = Registrar   BA = Barely adequate
SR = Senior Registrar   CR = Crowded   A = Adequate

two consultant units lacked refrigerators for storing blood, three units needed new mechanical ventilators, eight required additional calibrated vaporizers, and most units had no blood warming apparatus available in the theatre.

ANAESTHETIC SERVICES PROVIDED

We can now examine the actual rate of service provision in the various groups. During the survey period 4,469 items of anaesthetic service, as defined earlier were recorded. This corresponds to almost 1 service per 8 births; of these services, 291 were standby services, 1,578 were epidural procedures, and 2,500 were general anaesthetics.

In Table 2 we have set out, in the same group order by size as in Table 1, the measured anaesthetic workloads as revealed by the survey. The workload type is classified as either standby, epidural, or

TABLE 2

Anaesthetic service rates by group

Group	Total births (6 months)	Still birth rate 1,000 births	Standby rate	Total epidural rate	Total GA rate	Total service rate	Anaesthetic services recorded %
A	4,632	11·4	0·5	2·3	6·9	9·7	96
B	3,042	12·2	2·9	1·8	8·2	12·9	96
C	3,005	11·6	0·6	14·1	7·3	22·0	99
D	2,938	16·0	0	11·4	5·0	16·4	99
E	2,239	13·0	1·7	0·6	5·9	8·2	100
F	2,398	12·5	1·1	<0·1	7·0	8·1	93
G	1,904	13·6	<0·1	0·4	4·3	4·7	87
H	2,191	11·9	0	0	4·6	4·6	98
I	1,331	14·3	0·5	0	7·6	8·1	99
J	1,337	15·7	<0·1	0	6·2	6·2	93
K	1,740	12·6	0·1	0	7·1	7·2	94
L	1,161	17·2	0	0	5·9	5·9	88
M	1,200	13·3	1·0	1·2	6·5	8·7	98
N	1,230	10·2	0·4	0	5·3	5·7	96
O	1,171	6·8	0·1	2·9	9·6	12·6	100
P	1,009	28·5	0	0	4·1	4·1	98
Q	895	16·7	0·1	0	14·0	14·1	94
Regional average		13·1	0·7	3·0	6·7	10·4	97
Teaching group	2,465	22·3	2·6	28·7	11·4	42·7	98

All service rates are per 100 births.

other regional blocks, and general anaesthetics. These latter two classes include some patients who had both epidural and general anaesthesia performed separately during confinement. Only those services provided by anaesthetic staff are included, and these services are shown as rates per 100 total births in the group. The table also includes the total number of births during the survey period and the still birth rate per 1,000 total births. The last column gives the percentage of anaesthetic services for which detailed data was collected during the survey period. Since this table constitutes the main description of the anaesthetic workload which has been met by the available services, some observation and comments are necessary.

1. 'Standby' service

This service includes those circumstances in which an anaesthetic was not actually provided even though an anaesthetist was called, and occurs particularly in breech presentation and multiple pregnancies delivered vaginally. The table shows that this service varies throughout the region from 2·9 per 100 births in one group down to 0·1 or less in nine groups. In some groups a low or zero standby rate is accompanied by a high epidural rate and this is particularly true in groups C and D because, in the major hospitals in these groups, epidurals were used for breech and vaginally delivered multiple births in lieu of standby. In one group a very low standby rate is accompanied by a very high general anaesthetic rate and this may reflect obstetric policy or geographical circumstances. We believe that the standby rate may give the most sensitive index of total staff shortage since this service is probably the first to be abandoned when anaesthetic staff shortages are felt. If one considers that about 1 in 35 births are breeches and 1 in 80 multiple pregnancy, then the potential maximum standby rate is 4 per 100 deliveries. In addition if one assumes that one-third of these deliveries will be accompanied by general anaesthetic this would give an expected standby rate of about 2·7.

This hypothesis would then suggest that a total standby plus epidural rate of 0·5 or less, which is 12·5 per cent of expected maximum rate, could be interpreted as evidence of significant anaesthetic staff shortage. Nine groups all show low rates in this respect while that of group F is marginally low at 1·1 per 100 births. As we have suggested the result in group Q is complicated by the extremely high general anaesthetic rate and this may be related to the rarity of standby

services. Since almost one-third of all babies born during standby
services in this study were classified as depressed or subsequently died
the potential significance of a low or absent standby service rate on
the survival of the infant is obvious.

2. Epidural services

The distribution and availability of epidural services is even more
unequal. Eight groups provide none and three show very high rates
(C, D, teaching group). Epidural services are developing in six other
groups particularly as consultant anaesthetists interested in this
technique are appointed. It seems very likely that the demand for, or
interest in, this technique will grow, although a full assessment of
its potential place in obstetrics is beyond the scope of this document.
The data however do indicate the inequality of available services
throughout the Region and we suggest that this is related to inequality
in available allocated consultant sessions.

3. General anaesthetic services

The general anaesthetic rate varies considerably about a mean of 6·7
anaesthetics per 100 births with lowest rates 4·1 (group P) and 4·3
(group G) and highest 14·0 in group Q. There appears to be no clear
inverse correlation between epidural services and a low anaesthetic
rate which is surprising and requires further analysis. The caesarean
section rate is determined mainly by the obstetric practice in the
group and these operations provide the major indication for anaesthesia. In the majority of the groups this total section rate correlates
with the total general anaesthesia service rate and lies between 4·0
and 5·0 per 100 births with four groups providing notable exceptions.
When caesarean sections are excluded from the general anaesthetics,
and individual hospitals are considered, the three hospitals with very
high epidural rates, have general anaesthesia rates of 2·2, 0·7, and 2·2
while the non-caesarean section general anaesthetic rate averaged
over all obstetric units (excluding cottage hospitals and three hospitals above) was 2·8.

4. Provision of infant resuscitation by anaesthetists

Throughout the survey there are only four cases recorded of anaesthetists being called specifically to resuscitate an infant if they were
not already present doing standby, epidural, or a general anaesthetic
duty. This estimate may not be completely reliable but does agree

with the survey of paediatric help available at group hospitals in consultant units. Only one hospital of this type declared that paediatric help was not available, although in most units the paediatric help is usually of SHO grade only and in some units the paediatric unit was physically remote from the obstetric unit. The crude infant resuscitation rate for all procedures attended by an anaesthetist was 6·9 per cent although for individual service types these are:

standby 18·6 per cent   epidural 0·9 per cent

general anaesthesia 9·1 per cent.

The data disclosed in this study do suggest that much of the neonatal resuscitation at the emergency level is being provided by anaesthetists and this includes very junior grades of anaesthetist without experience as well as those at consultant level. We are unable to comment on the quality of this care.

5. Correlation with still birth rate

The still birth rate amongst all infants during the study period is also presented in Table 2. The scatter of results is considerable and we examined the possibility that this rate was related inversely to the caesarean section rate since this might reflect anaesthetic staff shortages and delays. There is certainly no clear linear relationship between the rates and this probably only reflects the multiplicity of factors which can determine still birth.

STANDARDS OF GENERAL ANAESTHESIA IN CONSULTANT UNITS

In this section we will examine the standards in patient care with respect to general anaesthesia in as much as they are revealed by our study. It is more useful to present this data by individual hospital rather than administrative groups and all the tables will show the results in this form.

1. Operational features

The chief indications for general anaesthesia were emergency caesarean section (41·4 per cent), elective caesarean section (26·9 per cent), forceps (5 per cent), repair of episiotomy or laceration (13 per cent), and placental removal (12·5 per cent). The most significant operational feature of the general anaesthesia associated with obstetrics is the large proportion of work which occurs as emergency procedures.

In our study 36 per cent of all cases occurred outside of the standard working day and this ranged from 20 to 48 per cent for individual hospitals. Coupled with this is the observation that, in more than half of all anaesthetics, the anaesthetist had less than thirty minutes notice of the anaesthetic while in 5 per cent there was a delay in commencement due to the anaesthetists' involvement in another case.

2. Assistance available for anaesthetist

One other important operational characteristic of obstetric anaesthesia which we wished to explore related to the assistance provided for the anaesthetist both during induction and at the termination of the anaesthetic. The assistant available was classified as none, untrained (either orderly or pupil nurse), trained nurse with special anaesthetic training, technician, or orderly with anaesthetic training and medically qualified.

Whenever more than one assistant was indicated, the most trained or qualified grade was counted. Since the anaesthetist is not only responsible for the care of his patient but frequently for the neonate as well, the assistance required for obstetric anaesthesia may have particular significance in determining safety. It is useful to look at the data in Table 3 where the assistant available at induction has been presented for individual hospitals. Untrained staff includes pupil nurses and orderlies while trained includes technician orderlies and certificated nursing staff.

There is a considerable degree of variation in the staff available; some hospitals rely heavily on nursing staff while others depend mainly on theatre technicians. Seven hospitals had more than 30 per cent of the general anaesthetics given with either no assistant or untrained help only at induction. It is particularly disturbing to note that in one hospital more than four-fifths of all cases of general anaesthesia occur with these circumstances. The data for assistance available at the termination of anaesthesia is similar to that given in Table 3.

As we have observed a large proportion of cases occurs after the usual working hours so that we also examined separately the position with respect to assistants for anaesthetists in those general anaesthetics which commenced after 5 pm or before 8.30 am. In general the situation at induction was similar to that seen when all cases were considered although the proportion of cases without assistants was distinctly greater in three units. Two of these consultant units are completely isolated from district hospitals and this undoubtedly contributes to theatre staffing problems. When the situation at the end of the anaesthetic procedure is examined, the availability of assistant

TABLE 3

*Assistant provided for anaesthetist at induction:
general anaesthesia (percentage)*

Hospital	None	Untrained	Theatre-trained orderly	Registered nurse	Medically qualified
I	3	16	41	37	4
II	0	5	74	7	14
III	1	4	1	83	12
IV	14	28	9	45	4
V	4	27	7	30	32*
VI	1	36	7	37	18
VII	0	10	32	35	23
VIII	12	24	0	54	10
IX	11	15	39	20	15
X	38	48	2	10	3
XI	4	12	41	12	31
XII	8	9	12	33	39
XIII	2	11	71	5	11
XIV	2	7	22	59	10
XV	9	22	3	45	20
XVI	10	19	7	64	0
XVII	1	1	87	3	8
XVIII	4	19	4	58	15
XIX	22	10	19	30	19
XX	11	18	4	39	29
XXI	1	2	80	14	4
Regional average	7	17	30	33	13
Teaching group	0	17	43	17	23

* Includes medical students.

staff is even more unsatisfactory; in six obstetric units there was no assistant available at the termination of the obstetric and anaesthetic procedure for 20 per cent or more of all cases.

STANDARD CARE: ANAESTHESIA FOR EMERGENCY
CAESAREAN SECTION

We will continue our assessment and comparison of maternity units by examining the management of general anaesthesia for emergency caesarean section. This procedure has been chosen, both because it is the commonest single indication for anaesthesia in obstetrics, as well as representing the conditions of greatest hazard with respect to the patient. The use of anaesthesia for a single standard obstetric procedure will then allow some additional comparisons between units. We will examine two indices of care:

1. Seniority (and hence the experience) of the anaesthetists.

2. The pre-anaesthetic preparation of the patient with respect to potential gastro-oesophageal reflux aspiration.

1. Grade of available staff

The staff grades responsible for the anaesthesia in cases of emergency section are presented in Table 4. The table also shows the number

TABLE 4

Anaesthetist's grade: emergency caesarean sections (percentages)

Hospital	Part-time clinical/medical assistant	SHO	Registrar	Senior staff senior registrar/ consultant	Allocated consultant sessions
I	2	31	48	19	2
II	1	0	52	45	9
III	0	37	57	6	2*
IV	0	4	94	2	1
V	0	54	37	6	1
VI	0	0	96	4	0
VII	19	11	11	59	3
VIII	0	26	51	24	0
IX	25	20	40	15	2
X	3	38	50	9	2
XI	9	40	29	23	0
XII	0	15	35	50	6
XIII	0	35	50	15	1
XIV	0	25	75	0	1
XV	61	11	21	7	0
XVI	5	0	90	5	0
XVII	0	0	82	18	1
XVIII	0	6	74	20	3
XIX	3	13	23	60	0
XX	0	73	20	7	0
XXI	2	58	31	10	0
Regional average	4	21	54	20	
Teaching group	1†	0	30	67	11

* Epidural sessions only.   † Trainee.

of allocated consultant anaesthetist sessions per week at the individual hospitals.

The data reveal an extraordinary degree of variation in work pattern. In four large consultant units less than 10 per cent of sections are anaesthetized by senior staff while in two of these units more than a third of these anaesthetics were administered by the most junior grade.

The smaller units show a similar pattern; in three units, half or more of all anaesthetics for emergency sections are administered by senior staff while in five others junior grades provide a third or more, and in another unit 61 per cent of section anaesthetics were given by part-time clinical assistants. If we classify all the hospitals into two groups with group 1 having three or more allocated consultant anaesthetic sessions and group 2 having less than three allocated sessions per week, we can perceive an important association. In group 1 hospitals there were 293 emergency sections of which 163 (56 per cent) were anaesthetized by senior grades of staff and 14 (5 per cent) by junior or part-time staff while in group 2 hospitals of 742 emergency sections, 101 (14 per cent) were anaesthetized by senior staff and 219 (30 per cent) by junior or part-time staff.

It is difficult to resist the belief that this association is causal and the significance of a sufficient concentration of specifically allocated consultant sessions becomes obvious.

2. Pre-anaesthetic preparation of the patient with respect to potential gastro-oesophageal reflux aspiration

Outstandingly the most important feature of the condition of aspiration regurgitation is the sequel to aspiration of acid gastric contents. It is known that, in the United Kingdom, approximately twenty maternal deaths are caused annually by this. It is fully appreciated that the chemical bronchopneumonia which defines the acid-aspiration syndrome results from aspiration of material with a pH of less than 3·0 and that if the aspirated matter is less acidic, the potentially lethal syndrome (Mendelson's) is much less likely to develop (1). During the past several years it has become part of the standard recommended therapy of labour to give antacids (usually Mag. Trisil, BPC, 15 ml given two-hourly) from the onset of labour until completion of the third stage. It is known that subsequent to a second dosage the pH of the intragastric contents will be raised above the critical level of 3·0. It is known to be unsafe to rely upon a single dose of antacid given, say, just before induction of anaesthesia for emergency obstetric surgery.

In an effort to prevent any regurgitation aspiration, cricoid pressure may also be applied to the patient by an assistant at the time of induction. This manoeuvre requires an informed and appropriately trained assistant and has become advocated as a further standard prophylactic technique during induction of anaesthesia.

We inquired at some length about the use of these methods during the survey and present now the results for patients having anaesthesia for emergency caesarean section. As with all the data there were marked differences between individual hospitals, ranging from some units where 100 per cent of all cases were given appropriate antacid therapy and cricoid pressure application, to units where only 20 per cent had received antacid and less than half were recorded as having cricoid pressure applied. To condense this considerable detail we will adopt the practice used earlier of presenting the results for the two classes of units. These results are seen in Table 5.

TABLE 5

Emergency caesarean sections (percentages)

Staff grade	Endotracheal intubation Group 1	Group 2	Cricoid pressure application Group 1	Group 2	Antacid therapy administered Group 1	Group 2
Senior staff	100	100	95	76		
Registrar	100	100	90	69		
SHO	100	100	100	81	94	58
Other grades (part-time)	100	100	40	47		

Group 1 hospitals: Consultant maternity units with three or more allocated consultant anaesthetist sessions weekly.
Group 2 hospitals: As above with less than three weekly allocated consultant anaesthetist sessions.

It is immediately obvious from the data in this table that performance in terms of the frequency of cricoid pressure application and antacid therapy is much better in group 1 than group 2 hospitals although we would only accept universal application of these measures as optimal.

As we have indicated earlier the cricoid pressure application is made by an assistant and these results do not indicate how effectively this manoeuvre is used. This depends on the quality and training of assistants and in general the use of trained assistants was more frequent in group 1 hospitals. The administration of antacid therapy is the responsibility of the nursing staff but the level of medical interest needed to maintain the automatic prescribing of the prophylactic therapy at ward level does require the active involvement of consultant anaesthetic staff in maintaining standards of care. The data in Table 5 and additional data relating to the blood matching status of these patients published elsewhere, demonstrate, we believe, the influence which consultant standards have on the anaesthetic practice of junior staff (3).

We would now like to turn to a consideration of obstetric anaesthetic practice in GP hospitals.

ANAESTHETIC SERVICES IN ISOLATED COTTAGE HOSPITALS
We will aggregate data from all cottage hospital obstetric anaesthetics to present some comment on obstetric anaesthesia in this setting.

In the Birmingham Region there are 23 hospitals of this category, containing 364 beds. Eleven groups contain cottage hospital beds and in some groups 35 per cent or more of all obstetric beds are so situated. During the six months of the survey 5,366 births took place in cottage hospitals and details of 38 general anaesthetics were recorded, giving a general anaesthetic rate of 0·72 anaesthetics per 100 births. This rate is only about 10 per cent of the rate recorded throughout the region as a whole, despite the fact that 15 per cent of all deliveries took place in these hospitals. This suggests that there is a high standard of discrimination applied to the selection of patients for cottage hospital obstetric care. Some features of these 38 cases are worth noting. As might be expected the majority of these cases were anaesthetized by GP anaesthetists and the commonest indications for anaesthetic were placental removal, repair of episotomy, or laceration. The recommended prophylactic therapy for gastro-oesophageal reflux-aspiration was incomplete, less than half the cases having been given antacid therapy, and cricoid pressure was recorded as having been applied during anaesthetic induction in only about one-third of the cases. Since half of these patients were not intubated or were difficult to intubate, this is a rather disturbing finding. Only three patients were matched for transfusion, while four cases had blood loss of more than 1 litre recorded.

Over-all the standard of service provided was not considered optimal and one case of Mendelson's Syndrome occurred in these 38 anaesthetics. The standard of equipment in several hospitals was poor, two hospitals even having deficient suction apparatus.

MORTALITY AND MORBIDITY

In the introduction to this report we stressed our interest in the experience of the authors of the confidential reports on maternal mortality. Although no inquiry of the type presented here can possibly determine fully the anaesthetic component of obstetric morbidity, it is important to make some observations about the problems associated with regurgitation aspiration for which the anaesthetist must usually bear full responsibility.

MORTALITY

During the survey period 5 deaths were notified in patients receiving anaesthesia; 4 of these patients received general anaesthesia and 1 had been given an epidural. In 3 of these cases no relationship between the anaesthetic and the death can be traced but in 2 cases, both cases of Mendelson's Syndrome associated with aspiration, the deaths are directly linked to the anaesthetic and this re-emphasizes the importance of this complication in obstetric anaesthesia.

Anaesthetic difficulties and complications

Regurgitation aspiration. In 22 cases of general anaesthesia gastro-oesophageal regurgitation with suspected or confirmed aspiration was recorded. In 9 of these cases the events were classified as major incidents since the patients were recorded as receiving a full measure of resuscitative therapy including endotracheal suction and steroid therapy. Two of these patients died.

The type of obstetric procedure, and the grade of anaesthetist involved, are detailed in Table 6. The data confirms the reasonable assumptions that the mishap is more likely to occur when the operative procedure is undertaken in haste, and occurs less frequently in the hands of an experienced anaesthetist. It must be noted well, however, that aspiration regurgitation does occur even at the start of a planned procedure, and is to be met with when the anaesthetist is of consultant rank.

The 22 cases of aspiration may be divided into two classes with reference to the grade of severity of sequelae. No ill-effects were observed either during or following the episode in 17 cases, including 5 in which cortisone and antibiotics were given as a prophylactic measure. Eleven of these patients (including 4 who received the appropriate intensive therapy) had more than one dose of antacid previous to anaesthesia; the remainder had received either no antacid (3 cases) or only one dose (3 cases): one of the latter received intensive therapy.

TABLE 6

The occurrence of aspiration regurgitation of gastro-oesophageal contents, related to the operative procedure and to the grade of anaesthetist involved. The appropriate prevalence per 1,000 general anaesthesias are indicated in brackets

Procedure		*Anaesthetist's grade*	
Elective section	3 (5·2)	Senior staff	4 (5·4)
Emergency section	12 (11·6)	Registrar	12 (11·0)
Pre-labour (excluding section)	2 (17·1)	SHO	4 (7·8)
During labour or delivery	4 (21·7)	Other	2 (18·3)
After labour	1 (2·2)		

Of the remaining 5 cases, 1 (no antacid) developed bronchospasm but rapidly recovered without treatment; 2 (one had had a single dose of antacid and the other had received, by the end of labour, only two doses) proved to be difficult to resuscitate; and 2 patients, neither of whom had been given antacid therapy, died, despite intensive therapy. These data may succinctly be expressed as follows:

	Died	Difficult resuscitation	Asymptomatic *No therapy*	*With therapy*
No antacid or only one dose (9)	2	1	4	2
Two or more doses of antacid (13)	0	1 (2 doses)	8 (one with 2 doses)	4 (one with 2 doses)

Also we can see that all 10 patients who received more than two doses were asymptomatic following regurgitation aspiration (including 3 who received intensive therapy) and of the 12 who received two or fewer doses, 2 died, 2 were difficult to resuscitate and 7 were asymptomatic (including 3 who received intensive therapy).

Four of the 22 cases of aspiration occurred in hospitals where there were at least 3 allocated consultant anaesthetic sessions, 2 received no therapy and were asymptomatic, 1 received therapy and was asymptomatic (these 3 had had more than two doses of antacid); and the fourth, who had received two doses of antacid before coming to emergency section after a failed forceps, proved to be difficult to resuscitate. The rate was 6 per 1,000 anaesthetics for group 1 hospitals and 10 per 1,000 anaesthetics for group 2 hospitals. The conclusion appears to be inescapable: a properly conducted regimen of antacid therapy is essential to the reduction in the rate of maternal mortality resulting from factors associated with anaesthesia. A further disturbing feature is that, as the two deaths which occurred were of patients undergoing caesarean section, the death-rate from acid aspiration associated with this operation during a six-month period in the Birmingham Region was 1·2 per 1,000, a figure to be compared with the incidence of 0·32 per 1,000 reported in relation to the same set of circumstances in the most recent, triennial *Report of Confidential Enquiries into Maternal Deaths (1967–1969)*.

It has been possible to present only a limited amount of data related to obstetric anaesthetic practice in this report and we would like to complete this paper by repeating our conclusions and recommendations as they followed from the more complete report.

Conclusions and recommendations

It is important to recognize that this study did not set out to prove that anaesthetics administered to properly prepared maternity patients by trained staff and assistants in a well-equipped theatre or labour ward are safer than those administered to inadequately prepared patients by untrained staff without assistance in ill-equipped or inappropriate surroundings. We regarded this as axiomatic and have attempted to use the data obtained during the survey to discover where and when the latter circumstances exist rather than the former, so that constructive recommendations could be made. The study revealed an excellent standard of obstetric anaesthetic care in some groups while in other units there was evidence of neglect with the existence of the unfavourable circumstances referred to above. We are convinced of the association between high standards, safety, and the employment of consultant anaesthetists with several allocated obstetric sessions. This is not to say that all units without allocated consultant sessions functioned inadequately. In some units dedicated consultant anaesthetists managed to maintain a high level of care but only under potentially difficult and often unacceptable conditions. The Birmingham Regional Hospital Board and its officers have recognized this association and there has been an increasing tendency to appoint staff with sessions specifically allocated to the obstetric units.

As we have suggested earlier it is impossible to divorce the question of staff anaesthetists from the way in which the obstetric service is itself organized and it is necessary to make some observations on the matter of obstetric bed organization.

ORGANIZATION OF OBSTETRIC BEDS

Quite clearly, it is manifestly easier to justify several allocated consultant sessions to a large maternity unit of 250 beds than to five such units each of 50 beds. Thus from the viewpoint of anaesthetic services, it is desirable to concentrate the obstetric unit service into large units. It is obvious however that in some parts of the country this will not be possible although every effort should be made to expedite closure of consultant obstetric units separated by several miles from the main district hospital services as a first priority. The birth-rate is falling and this should help to contain the total needs for obstetric beds at the present time.

The question of obstetric practice in cottage hospitals is a difficult one. We believe that cottage (or community) hospitals do have an important place in the over-all medical care strategy, but we do not feel their role in obstetric care is so clear. It is likely in the rural areas that cottage hospital maternity beds will need to remain but equally there are cottage hospital maternity units within easy and convenient distance of a consultant maternity unit and this seems hard to justify.

Our survey showed good clinical discrimination on the part of GP obstetricians as evidenced by the very low anaesthetic rate in the cottage hospital unit. The quality of the anaesthesia provided, as far as we can tell, was not optimal and if obstetrics is to continue in this setting some steps to improve the technical quality of the anaesthetic service should be undertaken. This will be referred to later.

STAFF

We believe that the key to uniformly high standards of obstetric anaesthesia depends on the appointment of consultant anaesthetists interested in the problems and the techniques of obstetric anaesthesia.

The Birmingham Region, for example, contains seven large maternity units of more than 110 beds and apart from the teaching unit, only one of these units has an anaesthetist with more than three allocated sessions. Most units have two or three consultants each contributing one or possibly two sessions weekly; in some cases these are limited to sessions for providing epidural analgesia. This is not, in our view, an effective way of obtaining good obstetric anaesthetic services. The consultant sessions should be concentrated so that they are the responsibility of one or two persons who each then may have three to five allocated sessions weekly, and the numerical justifications for this level of attachment is presented elsewhere (3). The importance of these consultants depends not only on their involvement in giving anaesthetics but probably more on their capacity to compete for suitable resident staff, and provide training and guidance for residents, midwives, and theatre staff. This sort of involvement will often arise out of self interest, which constitutes the most effective of all motives.

The large unit should have at least one full-time registrar seconded to it and one-half to one full-time senior registrar. In a large district hospital these positions can clearly be made part of a rotating residency. This pattern of staffing has been achieved on one unit at least and, we believe, it should be copied in the other large units. For smaller units is is clearly more difficult to justify this scale of staffing but our study has suggested strongly that *some* of these are short of staff at every level and that in these units there is real need for additional staff. Once again we would recommend a ratio of 3 allocated consultant sessions per 50 beds (1,500 births) of consultant/GP unit. Clearly this ratio will need to be modified by the over-all area distribution of beds and turnover since as we have shown in some groups a large proportion of beds exist in cottage hospitals. In regard to Junior Staff it is more difficult to provide a prescriptive recommendation but in general some additional registrar staff is certainly required in those groups where there is no standby service being offered at present. If our recommendation for consultant anaesthetists were applied throughout the Birmingham Region about 114 weekly sessions would be needed. At present there are already 26 such sessions in existence excluding the teaching unit. Thus the additional annual cost if all sessions were filled by new appointees (and this is probably unnecessary or unlikely) would be of the order of £50,000. It is more difficult to estimate resident staff increases but there is probably a need for two additional senior registrars and about ten registrar-grade anaesthetists, some of whom could replace SHO-grade staff or act as supports for this grade.

STAFF TRAINING

The quality and safety of obstetric anaesthesia depends on factors partly outside the direct control of the anaesthetist. The administration of antacid therapy is the responsibility of nursing staff; the application of cricoid pressure is the task of the anaesthetist's assistant. In some hospitals there is a shortage of any theatre assistant for the anaesthetist particularly at night and in others this assistant, if provided, is not adequately trained. We are convinced that one important role of the consultant anaesthetist with allocated obstetric sessions is to provide both the political force for rectifying shortages and the time and interest to train paramedical staff at ward and theatre level.

Our study has shown, as did Taylor's earlier postal inquiry, that in some units there is a heavy reliance on junior-grade anaesthetic staff. If for reasons of economy or staff shortage this is likely to continue then specialized in-service training in obstetric anaesthetic techniques and dangers should be provided for the junior anaesthetic personnel. This training should also be provided for GP anaesthetists and indeed could be made obligatory. This could help to enhance the present level of safety.

To provide all these components of training, it would be both economic and efficient to use the teaching hospital unit and three to four of the large regional maternity units in this special teaching role. For this purpose some small additional staff requirements might exist but if the region is to retain a significant number of small obstetric units this strategy could be useful both in raising standards as well as in making these appointments more attractive to the junior staff, and hence easier to fill.

This survey was made possible only because of the real interest and co-operation which existed in the Birmingham Region. It required the involvement of anaesthetists of all grades, midwives, and administrative personnel. The study represents an attempt at medical audit in a prospective setting and should be regarded as only a first step in the process of creating a uniformly excellent obstetric anaesthetic service. Such a service requires the co-operative efforts of several specialist groups as well as midwives and administrators and we hope that this study will provide a basis at least for evolving changes appropriate to the real needs and safety of the obstetric patient.

ACKNOWLEDGEMENTS
We would like to thank all anaesthetists who provided data on which the study is based and we wish also to express our gratitude for the considerable help received from midwives and nursing staff throughout the Region. Secondly, we must acknowledge the important contribution made by our three data supervisors, Mrs M. Flewett, SRN, SCM, Miss G. Shepherd, SCM, SRN, and Miss J. Richmond, SRN, SCM.

Lastly, we must thank the staff of Birmingham Regional Hospital Board for many items of assistance in addition to the financial support which enabled the study to be made.

References
1. BANNISTER, W. K., and SALLITARO, A. J. (1962). *Anesthiology*, **23**, 251.
2. CRAWFORD, J. S. (1970). *Br. J. Anaesthesia*, **42**, 70.
3. —— and OPIT, L. J. (1975). *Anaesthesia* (in press).
4. OPIT, L. J., and CRAWFORD, J. S. (1974). *Confidential Report to Birmingham Regional Hospital Board.*
5. TAYLOR, G. (1971). *Br. med. J.* **1**, 104.
6. —— and PRYSE-DAVIES, J. (1966). *Lancet*, **i**, 288.

J. A. Stilwell
MA
Health Services Research Centre
Department of Social Medicine
University of Birmingham

Christine Hassall
MSc, PhD
Department of Psychiatry
University of Birmingham

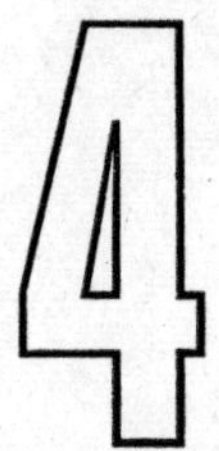

The evaluation of a new mental health care system :
Problems and approaches

The evaluation of a new mental health care system:
Problems and approaches

Introduction

It is more than a hundred years since the magistrates were empowered to set up 'asylums' to house what were then termed 'pauper lunatics'. In many parts of the country the system of care for the mentally ill is still based on admission to these same asylums. As these large hospitals are often sited in rural districts miles from the population centres in their catchment area, they are isolated from the communities they serve.

The past twenty-five years has seen the development of new concepts in psychiatry. New drug therapies and a growing feeling that long periods of stay in hospital could in themselves be harmful (1), lead to shorter (though often more frequent) admissions for all categories of patient. Psychiatric day care, started for the first time on an organized basis by Bierer in 1946 (2, 3), has become the preferred form of treatment wherever possible. All except the most disturbed patients or those who need the special facilities of in-patient care, can be treated for all or the greater part of their illness while living at home. Psychiatrists now believe that it is beneficial for most patients to maintain this link with home and family. Thus we are moving towards a new system of psychiatric care where the emphasis is transferred from in-patient beds to day places and supporting services, where the patient remains close to or preferably in his own community and home. Under this new community-based system there will be fewer beds and these will be provided in psychiatric units in district general hospitals (the main therapeutic centres of the changing Health Service) which should be more conveniently sited.

Parallel with this change of emphasis, and indeed essential if the new system is to function efficiently, supporting services such as day-hospitals, psychiatric hostels, group homes, domiciliary nursing and social work services are to be developed or augmented.

The DHSS decided to set up a full-scale community-based service for the mentally ill. This service will be used as a test-bed for similar services elsewhere. An old mental hospital will be run down and eventually closed: replaced by the creation of new beds and services as shown in Table 1. This new service has been planned to replace Powick Hospital whose catchment area of some 300,000 persons includes the City of Worcester and the greater part of the former county of Worcestershire. It is known as the Worcester Development Project.

TABLE 1

Now			Planned		
Name	*Beds*	*Day places*	*Name*	*Beds*	*Day places*
Powick	684	130	Newtown (Worcester)	150	160
St Wulstan's	*	*	Bewdley Road (Kidderminster)	60	80
			Malvern		20
			Evesham		20
			Worcester Day-Centre		40
			Group homes (Worcester)	6	
			Group homes (Evesham)	6	
			Kidderminster Hostel	12	

* St Wulstan's is a rehabilitation centre for the whole region.

The Worthing Experiment (4), the first well-documented excursion into community psychiatric care in this country, was started in 1957. Since this time it has become clear that commitment to the new type of service owes much to basic value judgements. Richard Crossman, the Secretary of State for Health and Social Services, said in Parliament on 11 February 1970: '. . . about one-third of the inmates (of mental hospitals), at a cautious estimate, could live outside hospital if provision were made for them. *They have to be brought out* because what they are suffering from is *rejection of society*' (5) (our italics).

Studies of the Worthing Experiment (6) have raised many interesting questions, and the DHSS decided to fund an independent research team to carry out an evaluation of the Worcester Development Project. This team was formed from members of the Department of Psychiatry and the Health Services Research Centre, of the University of Birmingham. Because many of the aspects of the studies at Worthing posed questions which bordered upon or were part of the economic branch of the social sciences, it was decided that there should be a specifically economic input to the research.

At the beginning of 1973 a psychiatric case-register was established for the Powick catchment area. This is a computer-based recording system which covers everyone who consults a psychiatrist (within the NHS) and records all the specialist psychiatric services they receive. This register has two main functions, to produce routine tabulations for those who provide the psychiatric services (doctors, social workers, etc.) and to provide a data base for the research team.

THE ROLE OF THE RESEARCH TEAM

'Evaluation' is a word with a ring of precision to it. A hypothesis is formulated, an experiment performed, the result evaluated, and the hypothesis accepted or rejected. Two preliminary conditions are necessary for the feasibility of this procedure. The first is that the object of the evaluation shall be defined. The second is that effective techniques of measurement should exist, and rules for the combination of measurements into indices. The less precise and less acceptable are the definitions of the object and the available techniques, the less appropriate is the concept of evaluation.

The problem of the identification of the role of the research team is exactly this problem; what is the range of the evaluation and what techniques can be used? Researchers in this field, aware of the difficulties, often avoid them by putting very strict confines upon the problems which they examine; for example people often wish to know if a particular therapy makes a particular patient or group of patients 'better'. In this context the word better is almost impossible to define satisfactorily. Instead researchers tend to ask specific questions like 'is he less depressed?', 'is he back at work?', 'is he managing without tablets?' Economics has developed the technique of cost-benefit analysis, where all the effects, or estimated effects, of policies are followed through, measurements made in terms of money, and measurements combined according to specifically stated rules, or weightings.

THEORETICAL PROBLEMS

The present job therefore requires an approach which is not customary to workers in the field of psychiatric research or economists. To evaluate a scheme of such size, to provide decision-makers with a clear-cut decision, or information in a clear enough and limited enough manner for them to make the decision, is foreign to the psychiatric research worker. The economist, accustomed to analysis where a conceptual distinction can be made between consumer, production function, and product, is thrown off balance when the consumer is not defined, and where, in many cases the product is itself part of the productive process.

The lack of definition of the consumer should not be a problem, but is. The answer would appear to be obvious: those at risk of mental illness or its effects; that is the people of Worcestershire. The Development Project, however, is intended to improve the response to the *demands made upon the specialist mental health services*. Effective demand is stated demand; the market price of soap is not affected by the unstated needs of the unwashed, but by the expressed demands of those who wish to be clean, and who know that washing is the way to go about it. Effective demand upon the psychiatric services is made by family doctors, not by patients. There are other channels for referral but they are quantitatively insignificant. A study, which we are starting for a number of reasons which we shall discuss later, is intended to estimate the adequacy of the planned provision of beds for those suffering from senile dementia. The adequacy of this provision has been questioned by local GPs and consultants, who are afraid that they will be unable to find places for some patients who they consider need admission.

It is, of course, perfectly proper to treat the expressed demands of family doctors as the basic demand variable (with, of course the implicit assumption that this is a good proxy for social need). This involves the standard economic assumption that the family doctor has a good knowledge of those of his patients who suffer from this condition, and that his demands upon the specialist services are not dependent upon his knowledge of the present, or some concept of a 'proper level' of supply of the services in question. Yet even given the satisfaction of these conditions, optimizing the number of beds available will only improve one aspect of the quality of life of those suffering from senile dementia, and this improvement may not be cost-effective; for example, greater benefits might be obtainable from the cost of the extra beds spent upon some form of home-based family support. (It may be interesting to note that the number of senile dementia beds planned for 1981 is 118 and according to the prevalence rates derived for Glasgow by Isaacs and Kennie (7) there would be about 950 cases. Direct extrapolation from Glasgow to

Worcester is not possible, but the orders of magnitude suggest that certainly the majority of cases of senile dementia will be maintained outside hospital.)

This is a theoretical problem of some magnitude in an over-all 'yes/no' evaluation. In fact, in practice, its importance is diminished in so far as the over-all nature of the evaluation is reduced.

The second theoretical problem is that economists are not accustomed to dealing with a situation where there is no distinction between a production process and a product and where a product itself is difficult to define. The economic models of the health industry, such as that described by Alan Williams (8), look at treatment as a cost incurring process (costs both to the health service and the recipient) with a desired output. It may be difficult to impute relative costs to acute and chronic pain, or to measure the benefits of increased life expectancy, but it is in principle a procedure which accords with economic conceptualization. Consider, however, the regime of psychiatric day-care. It is quite possible to find patients with similar conditions who have, and have not, had day-care, and whose end-state is similar. If day-care were a 'normatively neutral' procedure, such as industrial therapy, then, since it has a positive cost, it would be possible to suggest that it should be discontinued for this type of patient. Yet day-care is not necessarily expected to provide a 'cure', it is often the maintenance of a patient at a 'desirable level' for an indeterminate period. The same can be true of occupational therapy, where the use of the term therapy is sometimes somewhat loose. To take a second example, an enormous literature justifies nurse–patient contact in terms of the acceleration of recovery (9). A detailed study of nurse–patient interactions by Altschul (10) starts with a quotation, '[there should be a] broadening of the nurse's function in the mental hospital with the purpose of enhancing the therapeutic potential inherent in the nurse–patient relationship', and ends: 'In the writer's view, the most skilled performances observed were not in the realms of relationships, but in some of the interactions. The perceptive and sensitive way in which some nurses responded to patients' distress without any verbalization on the part of the patient was remarkable. . . .' Nowhere, however, was an operational hypothesis formulated, far less tested, which would enable the question 'What is the good of patient–nurse interaction?' to be answered, and clearly there is more to good nursing than the acceleration of recovery.

The development of standards,[1] whether general nursing standards ('pressure points every two hours'), broad quality of care ('all laundries in psychiatric hospitals to be equipped to clean or wash any type of linen owned by patients'), or medical standards ('each patient is to be examined by a medical officer as soon as possible after he is admitted') are a consistent response to the existence of qualitative scales (such as a scale formulated from the proposition 'the more nurse–patient contact the better') which resist quantification in a way which enables them to be combined with other scales. However sensible standards of care may be, they are in a sense anti-economic. The economist wants his functions to be continuous, not single points. He wants to be able to estimate the possibility of trade off between one service and another, and to arrive at an optimal combination of services. This process is undefined where the 'desirable' level of service is prescribed. Where the standard is a minimum standard, which may be exceeded, the situation in principle conforms closer to the economic model, but in practice the problem of attributing values to increments of the service may be great. In many economic evaluations, of course, these problems occur, but in few are they so central. Even if it is possible to arrive at a separate and operational definition of 'the product' it is commonly claimed that it cannot be measured, or if it can that it cannot be valued, or if it can that comparisons between values for two different people cannot be made. These are problems well known to welfare economics, and they do not, in fact, prevent cost–benefit analyses from taking place in other parts of the public sector, where benefits, such as time-savings (in, for example, the field of transport investment) are more amenable to expression in money terms than benefits in the health sector.

It has been asserted that the search for the definition of a product is futile: 'It has now become part of the economist's catechism that the NHS must be provided with some global numerical output function to interpret its financial data. We have serious reservations about the *need or the use* for such a measure, particularly as no output measure developed to date seems even remotely to provide a usable numerical index. The NHS has been steadily producing "output" since its inception even if we are unable to rationalize a numerical measure for

---

1. Performance standards in, for example, manufacturing industry are very different in nature. They are, or should be, standards designed to minimize the total cost of initial production plus the probable cost of rectifying faults.

it and there are many important financial issues in the management of the NHS for which the question of formalizing output is quite unnecessary' (11).

To the economist, however, this smacks of nihilism, and considerable effort is now being taken to devise systems of measuring output in order to escape from the '. . . intellectually imprisoning confines of the measures of workload and throughput (and even input) which too often are pressed into service as measures of the effectiveness of health care systems' (8), by devising systems of measuring output.

The difficulties surrounding the definition and measurement of output contribute to a further theoretical problem. Consider first the effects of persuasive (as opposed to informative) advertising on two sectors, first producers and second consumers. The effects on producers—for example, the installation by a manufacturer of a widely advertised air-conditioning system—can be evaluated with ordinary economic techniques, according to its effect upon the total costs of producing the factory's output. But the second, where consumers *are persuaded* that they want, and therefore they *do* want, particularly expensive after-dinner chocolates, presents enormous problems in the drawing of welfare conclusions from economic analysis. This problem was presented by J. K. Galbraith in 1965 (12) but the effect has been well known to the managers of psychiatric hospital services for a long time. For example, in a study of the psychiatric services in Plymouth, before and after the provision of a new psychiatric day-hospital Kessel and Hassall (1971 [13]) found that the new service appeared to have attracted a whole new group of patients. Now if bed stay is therapy (true production) then, in accordance with the arguments outlined above, no extra problems are presented. But if it is, at least in part, consumption (if it is the provision of a sheltered environment) then the automatic filling of a bed 'because it is there' becomes very difficult to evaluate.[1]

THE RESPONSE TO THESE PROBLEMS

These then are some of the main theoretical problems which stand in the way of a generally acceptable 'yes/no' over-all evaluation. The

1. This problem, of the interdependence of demand and supply, is endemic in the Health Service, and has made more difficult, among other things, the evaluation of multi-channel biochemical analysing machines (because clinicians often request tests merely because they are available) and central linen service systems (because ward sisters tend to use up whatever they are supplied with).

research team has, therefore, decided to approach its task in a different way, in one way more limited, in some ways more extensive. It is perhaps desirable to explain here what is meant by saying that in some ways the study will be more extensive. An evaluation of an experimental service is conventionally before and after, with and without. Measurements are made, and values assigned, to output variables before innovation, and the same done after the innovation, with appropriate adjustments for exogenous change. The net benefit is then compared with the net cost of the innovation. To take an analogy from a field where cost–benefit analysis is well established, a new type of roundabout might be installed in a road network. Traffic speeds and flows would be measured before and after the installation, time savings calculated, values of time imputed, and the savings compared with the cost of the roundabout.

The Worcester Development Project, however, is not simply a piece of capital investment. It is (or is intended to be) the physical and philosophical development and expression of a new idea, and as such is developing its own dynamic, dependent not solely upon the construction of certain buildings at certain specified times, but dependent also, and perhaps even more importantly, on the personal reactions and interactions of all those responsible for the many different elements which contribute toward the delivery of psychiatric care. We accordingly see one of the most important functions of the research to be the provision of monitoring information which will affect the course of the Development Project. An example of this is information about changing population estimates which may affect the level of provision of services. When the Development Project was initiated, the estimate of the 1971 population of those over the age of 65 was 34,930, and the estimate of the 1981 population of the same age-group 50,420. This growth was expected to depend on the ageing of those who migrated from the West Midlands conurbation in the late 1960s and early 1970s. In fact, the 1971 population of over-65s was 39,000 but the figure is not now predicted to grow to be as high as 50,000. This information could affect the timing of the opening and closing of beds for those conditions the incidence of which correlates with age: extra provision should be accelerated but may be slightly reduced in scale. (The standard provision of beds for the over-65s is 10 beds per 1,000 elderly people.)

If we now look back at the *simple* economic analogy which we made two paragraphs ago, we can see how badly it fits. In order to preserve the analogy, the road engineer would need to consult the economist about predicted traffic flows while the roundabout was under construction, and alter its design, or change its shape accordingly.[1]

In this sense, then, our work will be more extensive; it will be more limited in that it will attempt no over-all evaluation, but will instead concentrate first on separate studies of individual areas in order to avoid the problems of commensurability, and secondly on the provision of factual information intended to be of use to actual decision-makers.

We see, therefore, the primary purposes of the research to be as follows:

1. To predict the degree to which the physical and organizational elements of the Development Project will satisfy the demands set out in the Feasibility Report which was the departmental statement outlining the elements needed to provide a comprehensive mental illness service in the Powick catchment area (16).

2. To observe and monitor changes in *access to* and *methods* and *resource-costs* of care and to distinguish the four categories of change:

(*a*) Those independent of physical or 'philosophical' elements of the Development Project.

(*b*) Those dependent upon both elements of the Development Project.

(*c*) Those dependent primarily upon the physical elements of the Development Project.

(*d*) Those dependent primarily upon the philosophy of the Development Project.

To identify from 2 areas of unmet demand, or excess supply. These, if any, will result from estimation errors in the Feasibility Report, or from the emergence of types of demand unforeseen in the Feasibility Report.

---

1. Interestingly, the problem of interaction between evaluator and performer is well known in the field of social and psychiatric research, so much so that its own taxonomy has been developed (14, 15):

   Complete observer
   Observer as participant
   Participant as observer
   Complete participant

(The natural inclination of the present authors is for the first; but this just does not seem possible.)

3. To estimate the total costs of mental health care according to the distribution of those costs and their most significant determinants, and to monitor changes in the importance of these determining factors as the Development Project progresses.

The main research tool is a case-register, which was described at the beginning of this paper. This will provide data for many of the routine measurements ('monitoring indices') which will be produced on a six-monthly basis, but many of the monitoring indices require additional data the extraction and estimation of which are major studies in their own right.

PRACTICAL PROBLEMS

Three practical problems can be illustrated by examining one of the monitoring indices which appears innocuous and easy to assemble from existing data:

'Current aggregate public sector costs (excluding services provided by family doctors).'

The elements of this index are costs borne by: (*a*) the hospital service; (*b*) local authorities; (*c*) the DHSS.

The accounts of the hospital service are detailed. So are the accounts of the local authorities, and quite satisfactory in so far as local authority residential accommodation is concerned. With respect to the fieldwork of social workers, however, since social workers ceased to be specialized, after the Local Authority Social Services Act (1968) it has become impossible to infer from staffing levels the staff–client ratio where clients are being supported for psychiatric reasons. The case-register records contacts between social workers and registered patients, but there is no information about (*a*) the length of contacts, (*b*) the proportion of a social worker's case-load represented by work with registered clients, and (*c*) the proportion of 'overhead time' (writing letters, discussing cases, etc.) generated by the registered clients. In order to estimate this a detailed and time-consuming activity analysis study is necessary.

The local office of the DHSS holds all the information relating to Social Security payments to patients on the case-register and their families. At the moment this information cannot be released to the research team.

The importance of this should not be minimized. Omission of this element would lead to an underestimate of the costs of community-based care relative to institutionalized care if patients receive more in Social Security when at home than when in hospital: a reasonable hypothesis, which should be tested.

The provision, therefore, of what appears to be a piece of simple financial information, turns out to involve problems of data collection, statistical analysis, and ethical problems of confidentiality. These are, in general, three of the four main practical problems with which this work is confronted. The fourth problem is a theoretical one, not conceptual, like the problem outlined at the start of this paper, but nevertheless posing problems wider than, for example, statistical significance. This problem is that it is seldom possible to obtain control groups in any straightforward way—any use of the inferential method has to be somewhat devious. For example, consider the study of the day-hospital which we are conducting. A claim which has been intermittently made since the start of the day-hospital movement is that day-hospitals are cheaper than residential hospitals. In a sense this is almost certainly true: a week in a day-hospital is probably cheaper than a week as an in-patient, on the reasonable assumption that the cost of bed space and night services at the hospital outweighs the cost of ambulance transport to and from the day-hospital.[1]

This is not, however, the important question, which is quite simply: does the provision of a day-hospital reduce expected costs? Only a proportion of those in day care are maintained with no other service; out of a cohort of 41 patients who attended the day-hospital regularly for twelve months half made use of other psychiatric services during this time.

It is not possible both for ethical reasons and because the Development Project is not designed to be a series of experiments, to conduct a randomized controlled trial, monitoring and costing the total care profile of patients assigned or not assigned to the day-hospital. The method adopted, therefore, is (using the computerized case-register):

1. Select a cohort of day-patients.

2. Inquire from the consultant looking after the patient the method of care which would have been adopted in the absence of the day-hospital.

3. Select a comparable group with respect to: (*a*) diagnosis; (*b*) sex; (*c*) age; (*d*) start of alternative identified in (2) at same stage in case-history.

---

1. This in turn depends upon the assumption that the patient has bed space at home at zero cost.

4. Check group from 3 with consultant: return if necessary, to 3.

5. Monitor and cost the subsequent histories of patients in both groups.

This is a somewhat contrived procedure, with an unwelcome element of subjectivity. Nevertheless, it seems the best procedure that the circumstances permit.

Two additional problems arise from the nature of the Worcester Development Project. The time span for the Project is estimated to be about ten years. The research team plan to monitor the old, the changing, and the new service, and in addition to carry out many detailed investigations, such as questionnaire studies into facets of the problems of mental health care. It is assumed that all these studies will be comparative, that is before and after the new services are available. It is a tenet of research work in psychiatry that it is desirable that the same people should be involved in these studies for the duration of the work. In practice, however, this sometimes presents difficulties.

The research team is an independent team and as such attempts, as we said earlier, to adhere strictly to the role of observer. However the team cannot function properly without the goodwill and co-operation of those who provide (and receive) the psychiatric services. Thus, particularly as it is felt that the team should provide a service, there may be difficulties when requests are made for studies to be carried out, which are of interest to the care givers. The study of bed provision for senile dementia cases was requested by local medical practitioners. While the research team had planned such a study it was not scheduled to take place for twelve months, however, since local opinion deemed that this was an urgent problem, the study has been brought forward 'in response to popular demand'. We were able to do this as we are still in the early stages of our researches. Should a similar situation arise in twelve months time it is unlikely that time would allow us to accede to it, and carefully established relationships might be damaged.

CONCLUSIONS

The importance of the Worcester Development Project is that it not only makes explicit provision for the whole range of back-up services so necessary for the proper functioning of the general hospital psychiatric units, but also ensures that these services are developed in parallel with the bed provision they are intended to complement.

This paper discusses some of the problems, both theoretical and practical, which we have considered during the early stages of the research project. In making the decision to use the global approach only in so far as computerized monitoring techniques can be applied and focusing in depth on the main facets of the services it is hoped to overcome most of these problems and provide valuable information about existing, interim and new services.

References

1. BARTON, R. (1959). *Institutional Neurosis* (Bristol: John Wright and Sons).
2. BIERER, J. (1951). *The Day Hospital; An Experiment in Social Psychiatry and Synthoanalytic Psychotherapy* (London: H. K. Lewis).
3. FARNDALE, J. (1961). *The Day Hospital Movement in Great Britain* (Oxford: Pergamon Press).
4. SAINSBURY, P., and GRAD, J. (1962). 'Evaluation of treatment and services', in *The Burden on the Community* (Oxford University Press for the Nuffield Provincial Hospitals Trust).
5. *The Times*, 12 February 1970.
6. GRAD, J., and SAINSBURY, P. (1963). 'Evaluation of the Chichester mental health services', in Gruenberg, E. M. (ed.), *Evaluating the Effectiveness of Mental Health Services, Millbank Memorial Fund Quarterly*, **44**, 1, 231–78.
7. ISAACS, B., and KENNIE, A. (1972). *Symposia on Geriatric Medicine* (West Midlands Institute of Geriatric Medicine and Gerontology).
8. WILLIAMS, A. (1974). 'Measuring the effectiveness of health care systems', *Br. J. prev. soc. Med.* **28**, 3.
9. WORLD HEALTH ORGANIZATION REGIONAL OFFICE FOR EUROPE (1957). *Seminar on the Nurse in the Psychiatric Team* (WHO: Copenhagen).
10. ALTSCHUL, A. T. (1972). *Patient–Nurse Interaction* (Edinburgh: Churchill–Livingston).
11. OPIT, L. J., and CROSS, K. W. (1974). 'Comparing hospital costs' (correspondence), *Hosp. and Hlth Serv. Rev.* (May).
12. GALBRAITH, J. K. (1965). *The Affluent Society* (Boston: Houghton).
13. KESSELL, N., and HASSALL, CHRISTINE (1971). 'Evaluation of the functioning of the Plymouth Nuffield Clinic', *Br. J. Psychiat.* **118**, no. 554.
14. GOLD, R. L. (1958). 'Roles in sociological field observation', *Social Forces*, **36**, 217–23.
15. PEARSALL, M. (1965). 'Participant observation as a role and method in behavioural research', *Nursing Research*, **14**, 37–42.
16. DHSS (1970). *Feasibility Study for a Model Reorganization of Mental Illness Services*, MO(MI) 56 (London: HMSO).

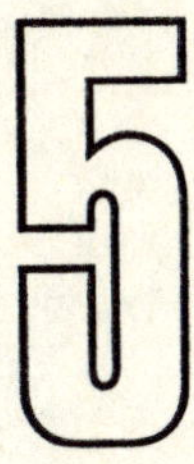

L. J. Opit
BSc, FRCS
Health Services Research Centre
Department of Social Medicine
University of Birmingham

P. R. Day
MRCS, LRCP, DOMS
St Mary's Hospital
Paddington

Regional hospital ophthalmic services. Suggestions for the comparison of available resources: their utilization, productivity, and outcome

Regional hospital ophthalmic services
Suggestions for the comparison of available resources: their utilization, productivity, and outcome

Introduction

Earlier authors have commented upon the inequality of resource allocation in the NHS (3). In a recent paper by Noyce, Snaith, and Trickey (8) attention was drawn to the positive correlation which exists between regional revenue allocation and the socio-economic status of the regions. These authors explicitly ignored any causal hypothesis for this relationship and in this paper we attempt to examine this in more detail using the ophthalmological hospital services as a model. Ophthalmology has been chosen because the hospital workload consists mainly of treating five well-defined classes of disease and of these, two groups, namely squint (strabismus) and cataract provide a substantial proportion of all admissions. These diseases are treated by methods which probably differ little from region to region.

We will attempt to compare the resources available in each region specifically for the hospital treatment of ophthalmic disease and suggest some simple comparative indices of utilization and productivity. To interpret even speculatively, these data, it is desirable to be able to compare regionally, the outcome which follows utilization of resources. This parameter, which in current management jargon is called the *output*, has no self-evident formal meaning in a medical service. In an informal sense it probably means the results of treatment, and for proper assessment, this requires an analysis of the therapeutic intention with respect to each patient and some qualitative measure of its attainment. It may well also include the patient's satisfaction with the service and even then we have only partially specified the output of an admission. At the present time a credible numerical analysis of this sort is impossible even on a limited scale and since our concern, in this study, is with large regional aggregates of patients we have adopted the assumption that for strabismus and cataract at least, output is equivalent to surgical treatment rates.

This assumes both the indications for treatment and the technical quality of the outcome of treatment are the same for all regions and thus completely ignore issues of technique, selection, and quality. It does, however, enable us to draw upon data already routinely collected and allows an exploration at least, of the potential uses of the vast body of data collected within the NHS, but seldom drawn together for analytic purposes. We are fully aware of the limitations of such an analysis but present it as an example of health service research which, even if it cannot provide unambiguous answers to the issues of resource and utilization, can at least direct attention to those questions which the administrative authorities and clinical services should themselves examine in more depth.

Method

Financial data used in this study has been obtained either from hospital cost accounts 1971/2 or by deduction from personnel data obtained from the DHSS (1972). Workloads for 1972 were obtained from the regional SH3 summaries and specific disease treatment rates from HIPE (1971). Regional population structure was that presented in the *Digest of Health Statistics* (1972).

Results

AVAILABLE RESOURCES

We commence our comparison of the regional ophthalmic resources by defining the primary resource inputs in two categories: beds and clinical manpower. These are presented in Table 1 for all regions in England. We have aggregated all the metropolitan regions together with the London teaching hospitals since there is known to be considerable inter-regional flow of patients and a very asymmetric distribution of beds, particularly in specialist ophthalmic hospitals situated in the metropolitan areas. The beds are expressed per million population and the adjacent columns show a further breakdown of these beds as proportions situated in previously designated board of governors' hospitals or in special ophthalmic hospitals (Type 18).

The clinician manpower is expressed in terms of salary payments as £s per 1,000 persons in the region and includes the costs of all hospital grades. The figure is not readily obtainable by direct means and has been computed by multiplying the number of ophthalmic hospital staff in WTE for each grade by the mid-point of the salary scale for that grade. Although some inaccuracy results from this estimation because it does not allow for different appointment age mixture at each grade, and will not include merit awards, it should provide a realistic standardization of available staff. Detailed examination of one region using both the measure and detailed local financial data suggests that this index is within 5 per cent of the true figure.

TABLE 1

Regional hospital resources for ophthalmology

Regional authority	Available beds per 10^6 pop.	Teaching hospitals %	Type 18 hospitals %	Clinical salaries per 10^3 pop. £s
Newcastle	94	0	19·9	56·6
Leeds	90	7·6	0	64·6
Sheffield	75	11·6	17·9	60·0
East Anglia	70	13·6	0	67·3
Metropolitan Region	105	39·5	8·5	77·0
Oxford	78	26·6	0	67·9
South-West	100	25·5	44·1	73·0
Birmingham	93	3·0	59·4	52·1
Manchester	94	38·4	0	54·8
Liverpool	105	54·7	0	45·8
Wessex	90	0	35	64·0
Average	94	—	—	64·9

An inspection of data in Table 1 shows two notable features:

1. Most regions have the same concentration of available ophthalmological beds, with three regions having reduced numbers of beds, and two having 10 per cent more than average. The location of the beds is, however, extremely variable; the Birmingham Region having almost two-thirds of the eye beds concentrated in five special hospitals while Leeds has its eye beds almost entirely distributed in acute general hospitals. These data presumably represent mainly the history of eye services inherited previously at the time of the NHS Act (1948).

2. The availability of clinicians to staff these beds is more variable from region to region than the availability of beds. Furthermore there is no correlation between the availability of beds and the distribution of clinical staff as measured by our financial index. Following the arguments of Noyce *et al.* (8) we have plotted the socio-economic index of a percentage of population in professional and management groups against the salary per 1,000 population for each region and

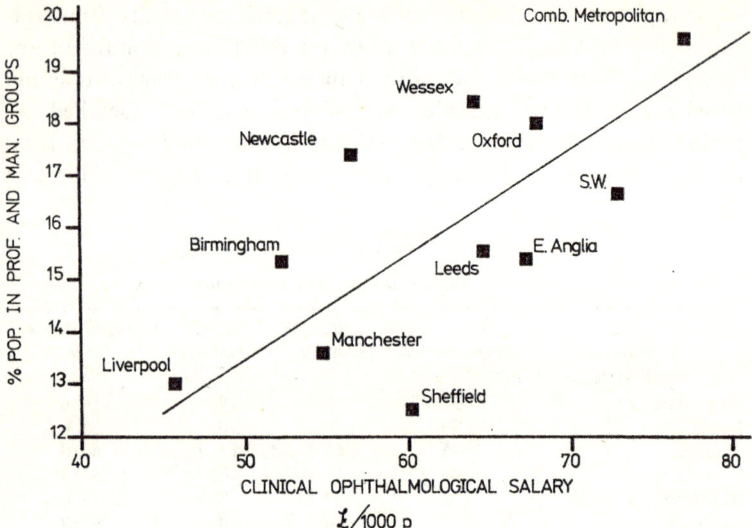

Figure 1. Plot of the proportion of households in professional and managerial groups against computed salary payable to all grades of ophthalmic clinical staff per 1,000 persons in the region.

this is shown in Fig. 1. The points lie around the line $X = 2 \cdot 6Y + 19$ ($r = 0 \cdot 74$) where $X =$ salary, $Y =$ percentage of professional and managerial staff in the region, and although the formal statistical correlation is not high it is difficult to escape the conclusion that some positive association exists between the employment of ophthalmic clinicians and the socio-economic status of the region. We are also now in a position to examine an earlier contention of Opit and Cross (9, 10, 11) that expenditure on therapeutic services and to a lesser extent on nursing are direct functions of the expenditure on clinical staff. Previously this had been examined using all acute services as provided in Types 1 and 2 hospitals. The presence of hospitals dedicated to ophthalmological services (Type 18) enables a more exacting test of this assertion to be made in one particular speciality by using the previously defined cost taxonomy and concentrating particularly in those regions where a substantial proportion of the eye services are provided in special ophthalmological regional hospitals. This analysis is presented in Table 2 where the therapeutic ratio is defined as the cost of all therapeutic and diagnostic services divided by the total clinical salary expenditure and the nursing ratio as total expenditure on nursing services divided by the total clinical expenditure. This method of analysis aggregates these costs for in-patients, out-patients, and operating theatres for reasons which are explained in these papers.

Only hospitals where a complete ophthalmological service, namely in-patient admission and surgical treatment as well as out-patient

TABLE 2

Cost ratios per unit clinical salary (£)

	Beds	Therapeutic ratio	Nursing ratio	Regional medical salary per 1,000 persons
Birmingham Region				
Average	219	1·28	1·17	£52·1
Hospital 1	103	1·28	0·80	
Hospital 2	98	1·30	1·75	
Hospital 3	18	1·12	2·73	
Wessex Region				
Average*	88	1·06	1·27	£64·0
Hospital 1	46	1·23	1·18	
Hospital 2	22	0·88	1·36	
South-West Region				
Average*	142	1·27	1·34	£73·0
Hospital 1	62	1·23	1·87	
Hospital 2	50	1·29	1·25	
Hospital 3	30	1·17	1·32	

* Some physiotherapy costs and X-ray costs missing.

department, are included since the mix of these components determines the final ratios. Some hospital cost account statements did not include a detailed breakdown of theatre costs and these costs have been distributed as medical, nursing, and therapeutic costs by using the average distribution from those hospitals where it was provided. The data in Table 2 suggests that the diagnostic and therapeutic demand for resources created by the ophthalmological services lies close to £1·25 per £1 of clinician salary even when there is a considerable degree of variability of the clinical salary itself. If only hospitals over forty beds are considered then the therapeutic ratio varies very little about 1·25 and suggests that this may be used as a good estimate of the cost of the use of therapeutic services by ophthalmologists.

The nursing ratios in Table 2 show considerably more variability and this is probably related to an assumption that the nursing staff allocation tends to depend both on the existing bed stock, the actual workload, and the relative proportion of in-patient to out-patient work. No obvious explanation exists for the wide degree of variation in the ratio. For example, the 100 per cent variation in the nursing ratio which is found in the Birmingham Region between Hospitals 1 and 2 is not explained by bed size or relative out-patient department/in-patient workload and it is tempting to speculate that either Hospital 1 has too many doctors relative to nursing staff or Hospital 2 has too many nurses relative to its medical staff. This marked degree of variation obviously needs further inquiry to determine the optimal ratio and to explore systematically the factors which should be considered as weights.

If our hypothesis that the consumption of resources by specialist clinicians in pursuance of their task can be expressed as stable function of the number of doctors involved, then the key measures of resource availability simply become the bed stock and the clinical staff density expressed as money units per 1,000 population. It now becomes relevant to attempt a comment upon the utilization of these resources.

THE UTILIZATION OF AVAILABLE RESOURCES
We would now like to examine the use of the two primary resource components defined earlier.

1. Bed stock
Occupancy rates of most ophthalmic units are low (60–70 per cent) and this is probably associated with a considerable load of short-stay cases, for example children with strabismus, who are treated during the week and discharged at weekends. It is useful therefore in discussing bed stock, to compare the queue of cases awaiting treatment as measured by the waiting-list size and express this as 'bed deficiency' per million population. This is easily achieved by dividing the waiting-list size by the case throughput per bed in each region. This measure assumes that:

(*a*) There is relatively little emergency admission work.

(*b*) The waiting-list case mix is similar to the treated case mix.

Both these assumptions seem likely to be valid with the ophthalmological waiting-lists. These results are shown in Table 3 by the regions using 1972 SH3 data. The relationship of this computed deficiency to the current available bed stock suggests one region at least is relatively deficient in available beds. The interpretation of the bed deficiency does require knowledge of the throughput or average bed occupancy. This will be presented later when considering individual case types since this will remove problems associated with different case mix.

TABLE 3

Bed usage and waiting-list size

Regional authority	Computed bed deficiency* per 10^6 pop.	Average occupancy rate %	Relative bed deficiency† %
Newcastle	14·6	61	15·5
Leeds	13·3	70	14·9
Sheffield	16·5	69	21·9
East Anglia	21·8	60	31·2
Oxford	14·7	63	19
South-West	25·9	60	25·8
Metropolitan Region	19·8	66	19
Birmingham	22·9	66	24·7
Manchester	21·3	68	22·6
Liverpool	23·2	61	22·2
Wessex	18·2	57	20·3
England	19·5	65	20·7

$$* \text{CBD} = \frac{\text{Waiting-list size}}{\text{Bed turnover number}}$$

$$\dagger\text{Relative bed deficiency} = \frac{\text{CBD}}{\text{Available beds}} \times 100.$$

2. *Medical manpower*

The assessment of the utilization of the other primary resource, medical manpower, is more difficult to present.

To achieve this we will adopt a strategy used previously in which an attempt was made to standardize the salaries by workload using a completely empirical approach (11). This depends on assuming that the medical salaries are a linear function of the number of new in-patient cases and new out-patient consultations, each treated as independent and this relationship is sought empirically by 'best line fitting' procedures.

To do this, we start by using the regional SH3 data as a basis for workload or case throughput although these data do not contain any measure of ophthalmological casualty cases. This can be obtained for individual Type 18 hospitals but is so variable from hospital to hospital that it is not possible to deduce what case-load exists in the region as a whole. One other problem exists with respect to the workload data on SH3 summaries and this relates to work classified as day cases. Nationally, the ratio of day cases to discharges and death is 12 per 100 and in six regions the ratios lie between 10 and 16 per 100. There are two regions with exceptional ratios: Liverpool, which has a very large number of day cases (43 per 100) and Manchester (4 per 100) which has very few. There is no obvious explanation in terms of either beds or clinical salaries for the state of affairs and we considered that the most plausible explanation is that the difference in numbers of day cases is due to variation in classification rather than case types. Since we wished to standardize the clinical salary for each region against the reported workload by empirically finding the best line which fitted the workload data and salary data, it was necessary to examine several hypotheses with respect to the day cases. We used the following assumptions:

(*a*) Day cases were different from in-patient cases and should be treated independently.

(*b*) Day cases were the same as in-patient cases and should be added into these data.

(*c*) Day cases were similar to new out-patient cases and since the number was small relative to out-patient numbers, these could be added to the new out-patient cases.

Two fitting techniques were used for each hypothesis:

(*a*) The total deviation between actual points and the fitted line should be minimized, the standard multiple linear regression procedure.

(*b*) The deviation between points and line should be minimized with respect to maximum deviation at any point (1).

After obtaining the best line for each hypothesis, the predicted salary was calculated from the coefficients of the line and the workload data. The predicted salary so obtained was divided by the actual salary for each region and was normalized so that national average had ratio 1. This statistic is referred to as the *normalized productivity ratio* and gives a standardized financial measure of the workload. If the ratio is greater than 1 for a region it expresses the assumption that the case throughput by ophthalmological clinicians in that region is greater than average for a given salary expenditure on ophthalmologists. Conversely a ratio less than 1 implies that the case throughput is less than average, given the work force expressed in salary expenditure terms.

In Table 4 we have presented the results of this analysis for the most likely hypothesis, namely, that day costs can be treated as new out-patients with the point wise fitting technique and we have ordered the regions under the hypothesis from highest 'productivity' downward. The data analysis shows that most regions are within 10 per cent of the national average for productivity. Sheffield, Wessex, and

TABLE 4

Clinical productivity

Regional authority	Predicted salary* for workload per 1,000 pop. £	Actual salary per 1,000 pop. £	Normal productivity
Birmingham	63·0	52·1	1·29
Liverpool	49·9	45·8	1·16
Oxford	71·3	67·9	1·12
South-West	73·0	73·0	1·06
National average	61·0	64·9	1·00
Combined Metropolitan	71·6	77·0	0·99
Manchester	48·8	54·8	0·95
Leeds	56·2	64·6	0·93
Newcastle	47·5	56·6	0·90
Sheffield	49·8	60·0	0·88
Wessex	52·5	64·0	0·87
East Anglia	54·5	67·3	0·81

* Predicted salary (pointwise fitting with zero intercept) $= 3·55X_1 + 3·94X_2$ where X_1 = discharges and deaths and X_2 = day cases + new out-patients.

East Anglia are the least 'productive' while Liverpool and Birmingham have a productivity which is considerably higher than average. If the hypothesis about day cases is changed there is little alteration in the ordering of productivities, nor is the order changed much by using multiple regression technique to carry out the fitting procedure. When the data in Table 4 is compared with that in Tables 1 and 3, it is tempting to hypothesize that the low productivity of Sheffield and East Anglia may be associated with a shortage of ophthalmological beds (although not of clinicians) and the high productivity of Birmingham is associated with the efficient use of ophthalmologists by ophthalmological service organizations in that region.

3. The use of paramedical staff
The situation in the Liverpool Region is mysterious and the reasons for large numbers of day cases when there are plenty of beds and the

lowest density of ophthalmological staff in England, are not obvious. The utilization of medical manpower in the eye services is complicated by the use of trained paramedical staff as a possible substitute for doctors, to do certain examinations such as sight testing or refraction, field plotting, tonometry, and orthoptics. This work may be performed by medical staff or paramedical staff and the pattern of

TABLE 5

Paramedical workload

Out-patient attendances at optician and orthoptic clinics expressed as number of attendances per year per £1,000 clinical medical salary in each region

Region	Attendances per £1,000 medical salary
East Anglia	192
Wessex	204
Newcastle	272
Leeds	280
South-West	303
Manchester	362
Sheffield	367
Oxford	454
Liverpool	510
Birmingham	521

work sharing will clearly affect the outcome of the productivity index as it is applied to clinical ophthalmological medical staff. In Table 5 we have expressed the workload of the paramedical staff in each region as the numbers of out-patient attendances at optician and orthoptic clinics as a function of the numbers of available doctors (in financial terms). There is a threefold range in this ratio across the regions, which does indeed suggest a considerable difference in either the use or availability of paramedical staff, and it will be noted that this order is almost the reverse of that seen with productivity indices in Table 4, so that a plot of these parameters against one another gives a good approximation to linearity ($r = 0.93$). We would interpret this as meaning that one important factor which determines a higher productivity index for clinical staff is the increased use of paramedical staff for out-patient work.

REGIONAL OUTPUT: SURGICAL TREATMENT RATES

As we have suggested earlier, it is reasonable in the first instance to regard the output of the hospital ophthalmic services as equivalent to the treatment rates of specific eye conditions and we will examine this contention by considering two common conditions namely strabismus and cataract.

Strabismus

Squint is a relatively common affliction probably affecting 6–7 per cent of all children under 5 years. The treatment can be conducted at out-patients but may require admission for surgical correction at some stage. By the use of *HIPE* data it is possible to compare the surgical treatment rates for this condition by region and relate this both to the availability of staff and socio-economic characteristics of the region.

In Fig. 2 we have plotted the corrected surgical treatment rates by hospital ophthalmic salaries for the regions. The corrected rates are computed assuming that the proportion of cases under 15 is the same for each region and equals the proportion in the national data. This proportion of treatment cases for each region is then divided by the population under 15 years in that region and the rate is expressed per 100,000 persons under 15 years. The figure suggests that there is a positive association between increasing treatment rates and regional clinical ophthalmic salaries with a surprising range in treatment rates from Liverpool (150) to Wessex (300). A similar distribution occurs if case rates are plotted against regional socio-economic status with the Wessex region showing a very high treatment rate both in relation to salary and socio-economic status. In Table 6 we have set out the average in-patient stay for cases with squint (1971). The data show a twofold range and generally these average lengths of stay show a negative association with the socio-economic status of the regions. In a region such as Oxford it is possible to treat two children per week in every bed whilst in Sheffield or Liverpool only one such child could be treated.

Cataract

Equally important as a major component of ophthalmological work load is cataract. Once again the *HIPE* data has been used to standardize surgical treatment rates per 10,000 persons over 65 years for each region and these data are also plotted in Fig. 2. The points are

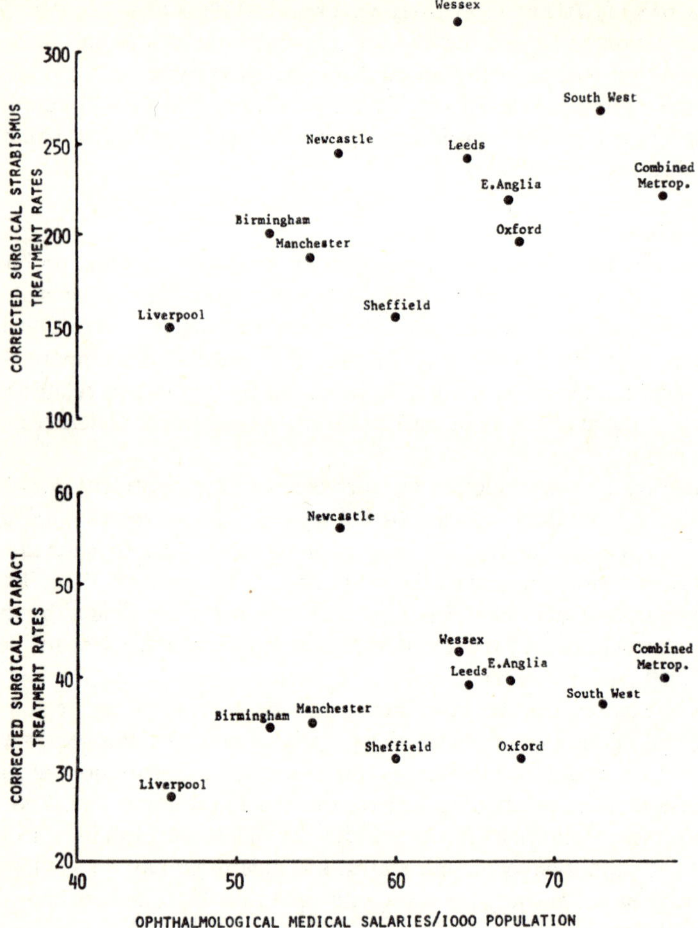

Figure 2. Plot of corrected surgical treatment rates (standardized for age) for strabismus and cataract against salary payable to all grades of ophthalmic clinical staff per 1,000 persons in the region. Treatments for strabismus: per 100,000 persons over 65 years. Treatments for cataract: per 10,000 persons under 15 years.

clustered around a line of positive slope with only one point diverging markedly from this line. This point corresponds to the Newcastle Region which shows an extremely high cataract rate, being more than double the rate in the Liverpool Region. A similar appearance is produced if the salary ordinates are replaced by regional socio-economic indices.

The length of stay for cataract cases is also available in Table 6 (1971). There is once again some negative association with socio-economic regional status. The length of stay in the Newcastle Region is only two-thirds of that in the south-west although these regions

TABLE 6

Duration of stay for cases of strabismus and cataract

Regional authority	Households in professional and managerial grades %	Average stay Strabismus (1971) (days)	Cataract (1971) (days)
Combined Metropolitan	19·4	4·0	13·2
Wessex	18·4	2·9	10·6
Oxford	18·0	2·6	12·1
Newcastle	17·4	3·2	10·2
South-West	16·7	4·6	15·0
Leeds	15·5	4·2	13·0
East Anglia	15·4	3·1	12·6
Birmingham	15·3	3·8	13·6
Manchester	13·6	3·8	12·7
Liverpool	13·0	5·6	12·9
Sheffield	12·5	5·1	14·3

have similar proportions of social class I and II households. This may be associated with cataract extraction carried out at an earlier age in Newcastle. It should be observed here that there is an increasing tendency outside the United Kingdom to reduce the length of stay for cataract extraction to one week or less and early discharge is now regarded as a safe procedure (14).

The association between length of stay, socio-economic status, and treatment rates is complex. On the one hand pressure of work (high treatment rates) reduces length of stay and on the other hand early discharge will probably be safer and easier to obtain with patients from social class I or II environments. The average length of stay data may also now be compared with data relating to the waiting-list queue, in Table 3. Thus the high computed bed deficiencies in some regions such as the South-West Region, well endowed with beds and clinicians, may be related to long average stay. Conversely in the Newcastle Region there is a rapid throughput of cataract cases in spite of a relative deficiency of clinicians (compared with average).

Taken together these data indicate a considerable range in the surgical treatment rates of the two commonest eye conditions, one predominantly a disease of children and the other afflicting mainly the aged. In general the 'poorer' regions have the lowest treatment rates and longest lengths of stay while the richer regions have the highest rates and shortest average lengths of stay although the associations are not monotonically linear using the usual orthodox statistical assumptions.

Discussion

In the data analysis which has been presented, we have tried to examine the regional ophthalmic specialist services by comparing both the primary resources available (beds and clinicians) and the way in which these resources are used. In such a broad and simplified analysis conclusions must be guarded; nevertheless, certain features seem worthy of comment.

1. The availability of beds and clinicians do not appear to be correlated. Three regions have significantly less beds than the majority while there is some association between clinicians available in money terms and the socio-economic status of the region.

2. We have used the waiting-list size and bed turnover to estimate a 'relative bed deficiency'. Although this is highest in the region with the lowest number of beds per million population, the computed relative deficiency does not suggest that there is any bed shortage in the majority of the regions and that variations in waiting-list size may be related to the average length of stay.

3. The use of the clinicians' services is estimated by a 'productivity index' with various assumptions. On this basis, the majority of regions have the expected average productivity with four regions displaying significant divergence. Two of the least 'productive' regions are those with the lowest bed numbers (East Anglia and Sheffield), while one region has a persistently high productivity (Birmingham). This region is exceptional in that two-thirds of all ophthalmic beds are in specialist hospitals. The productivity indices for the regions seem to vary directly with the amount of hospital out-patient work delegated to paramedical ophthalmic staff.

4. One other region which shows high productivity (Liverpool) has an exceptionally large number of day cases in spite of having the highest bed numbers and the lowest clinical salary per unit population and this may affect the results of our productivity analysis.

5. The expenditure on therapeutic services by ophthalmologists seems to be a function of the number of ophthalmological clinical staff and the ratio of expenditure is close to £1·25 per £1 ophthalmological clinical salary. The expenditure on nursing services expressed in this way is much more variable and no functional explanation is apparent.

6. If the surgical treatment rates for cataract and squint are regarded as measures of output albeit without qualitative judgement, it becomes possible to hypothesize further about the causes and effects of the varying resource mix and its utilization.

In general the possible relationships between resources, their utilization and surgical treatment rates are complex and interactive. Three possible but not exclusive factors could be surmised.

(*a*) Increased hospital referral for the treatment of squint and cataract increases the demand for more resources, particularly clinical staff. Increased referral rates might reflect a higher prevalence of the disease, increasing expectation of a good outcome from treatment or increasing awareness of the conditions by patients or their family doctors.

(*b*) The existence of specialist eye hospitals, dating before the NHS Act may have determined the distribution of ophthalmologists and this in turn has created the level of possible utilization without respect to need or disease prevalence. The growth in revenue allocation for the NHS has tended to maintain this previous hierarchy of allocation and this may have been related to socio-economic factors within the country. In simple terms those areas with many ophthalmologists, particularly professionally prestigious ones, have increased their numbers at least as extensively as the areas which had few and these staff levels have determined the treatment rates.

(*c*) For any given referral rate of cases the demand for clinical staff has depended on the productivity of the existing staff and this has been a function of the particular regional organization of ophthalmic services. It is worth examining these issues for the two main diseases separately.

STRABISMUS
There have been a number of prevalence studies of this condition (2, 15) which suggest that prevalence lies between 6 and 7 per cent for child populations under 5 years of age. Two potential factors which might influence the prevalence have been suggested. The first of these

is genetic although the available data would require a complex multifactorial genetic effect. The second factor follows from the observations of Miller *et al.* (6), which is not supported by later epidemiological work (2), showing a correlation between the prevalence of squint and deficient height, defective domestic environment and hygiene. This could infer that the prevalence of squint itself might be correlated negatively with increasing socio-economic status in the regions. The surgical treatment rates, however, show a positive correlation with this factor and an explanation for the surgical treatment rates based on other factors must therefore be considered. There is good evidence that the demand for services in general practice is higher from persons of social classes I and II than from persons from social classes IV and V and this occurs particularly with the children of such families (5). If the general level of demand for specialist eye services is raised by such a mechanism it will, in turn, gradually lead to an increase in the number of clinical ophthalmological posts required to meet this demand. The actual divergence in treatment rates for strabismus between say Sheffield and the metropolitan regions is probably even greater than that expressed by the data in this paper since it neglects the cases treated privately and this should again correlate positively with the general socio-economic status of the region. Some support to this contention is obtained by computing the average number of NHS sessions per consultant for each region.

One other factor may influence the surgical treatment rate for squint as distinct from prevalence and this is the availability of alternative non-surgical therapy. Since the conservative treatment of squint requires trained paramedical personnel the shortage of these personnel may effect the surgical treatment rate. This possibility is difficult to examine indirectly by workload data. A recent survey by the British Orthoptic Board does show a considerable variation in the numbers of orthoptists by region but there does not appear to be any consistent relationship between these numbers and the surgical treatment rate of squint (13).

CATARACT

Studies of elderly persons at home suggest a high cataract prevalence of about 15 per cent (4) although clearly this is not the prevalence of cataract suitable for treatment. The prevalence of cataract increases steeply with age and hence will be sensitive to the age profile. The data available in the *HIPE* only gives the prevalence of treatment and this introduces a significant difficulty. Senile cataract is usually a bilateral disease and we have no knowledge from *HIPE* sources of the number of cases per region having one or both eyes treated. The treatment of the first eye is probably highly effective from a cost-benefit viewpoint and the treatment of the second eye much less so (12). The inclination to treat both eyes may be related to socio-economic factors or to the beliefs of individual ophthalmologists and variations on this may partly account for some regional differences. The Newcastle Region has had a persistently high cataract treatment rate from 1965 to judge from *HIPE* data and this seems to be in excess of what might be expected solely from the socio-economic structure of the region. We are unable to determine whether regional differences are due to variations in prevalence, in awareness of defective vision, in anxiety concerning hospitalization, in knowledge of the benefits of extraction, or in the enthusiasm of ophthalmologists for a perfected surgical procedure.

One possible aetiological factor which could increase prevalence in some regions is industrially produced cataract associated with heat exposure in the glass and steel manufacturing industries (7). A recent paper has suggested that even the lens opacities of the type not usually associated with heat exposure are more common in workers in these industries than amongst a control population (16).

We must conclude therefore, that differences in disease prevalence do not account for major differences in surgical treatment rates. If the treatment rates for strabismus and cataract are accurate and if the effect of private practice can be ignored, we are left with the belief that the inequality of resource allocation is in part at least, the result of inequality of the demand for ophthalmological hospital services rather than vice versa. In crude terms, this means that in the Liverpool or Sheffield Region only half those cases of squint which would be deemed as requiring surgical treatment in Wessex, are being referred to ophthalmological services for treatment. This in itself will help to determine the available ophthalmological service since it is probably the pressure of demand created outside the administrative apparatus of the NHS, but ultimately transmitted through it, that has, in the past, determined some of the priorities of resources allocation. If, as we believe, these differences in resource allocation do express regional differences in the standards of eye care, the most important corrective step may be in the areas of patient or GP education and staffing in the community services rather than in the hospital-based eye services. The average cost at 1972 prices of clinical ophthalmologists of all grades is £64,000 per million population and this would represent (at 1972 prices) six consultants, two senior registrars, three registrars, and four house officers. It is difficult to estimate *a priori*, the actual requirements for ophthalmic clinicians although the average in-patient case-load for ophthalmic consultants is low when compared with that in, say, general surgery and ortho-paedics. On the basis of need currently being met by the services, there would appear to be an adequate level of staffing for in-patient services. While in-patient work calls for surgical skills, out-patient work calls mainly for medical and optical skills and the adequacy of provision may then depend on the way in which services are organized.

Our findings indicate that some regions, in spite of a relative shortage of ophthalmic clinicians, have obtained a high productivity, possibly, by a more extensive employment of paramedical staff. This may have arisen because the heavy case-load of optical and orthoptic work in the eye services has been met by the paramedical staff enabling the expensive medical skills to be reserved for clinical work appro-priate to those skills. If this is so, and the practice does not entail lowering of clinical standards, then the resources needed to meet present and even future loads, may be achieved in some regions by a modest additional investment in paramedical staff.

This, of course, assumes that conditions can be made attractive enough to recruit such staff. In regions already well endowed with ophthalmic medical staff the prime need may well be a concentration and reorganization of in-patient services and the development of community-based out-patient services for those patients who do not require hospital facilities.

References

1. BARTELS, R. H., and GOLUB, G. H. (1968). *Comm. A.C.M.* **11**, 428.
2. GRAHAM, P. A. (1974). *Br. J. Ophthalmol.* **58**, 224.
3. GRIFFITHS, D. A. T. (1971). *Hosp. and Hlth Serv. Rev.* **67**, 229.
4. HOBSON, WARD, and PEMBERTON, J. (1955). In *Health of the Elderly at Home* (London: Butterworth).
5. MARSH, G. N., and McNAY R. A. (1974). *Br. med. J.* **1**, 319.
6. MILLER, F. J. W., COURT, S. D. M., WALTON, W. S., and KNOX, E. G. (1960). In *Growing Up in Newcastle upon Tyne* (London: Oxford University Press).
7. MINTON, J. (1949). In *Occupational Eye Diseases* (London: Heineman).
8. NOYCE, J., SNAITH, A. H., and TRICKEY, A. J. (1974). *Lancet,* i, 554.

9. OPIT, L. J., and CROSS, K. W. (1973). *Hosp. and Hlth Serv. Rev.* **69,** 44.

10. —— —— (1973). *Br. med. J.* **4,** Suppl. 13.

11. —— —— (1973). *Hosp. and Hlth Serv. Rev.* **69,** 254.

12. PHILLIPS, C. I. (1973). *Lancet,* **ii,** 33.

13. BRITISH ORTHOPTIC BOARD (1969). Report. Unpublished data.

14. STRACHAN, I. M., and BOWELL, R. E. (1972). *Trans. Ophthalm. Soc. U.K.* **92,** 629.

15. THOMSON, E. (1922). Ibid. **42,** 273.

16. WALLACE, J., SWEETNAM, P. M., WARNER, C. G., GRAHAM, P. A., and COCHRANE, A. L. (1971). *Br. J. of Ind. Med.* **28,** 265.

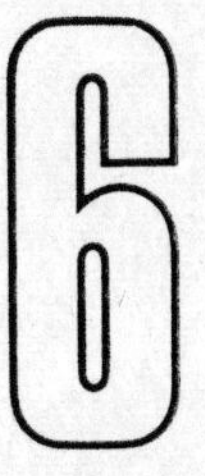

Susan Shaw
SRN
Health Services Research Centre
Department of Social Medicine
University of Birmingham

The role of the nurse in assessing the health of elderly people

The role of the nurse in assessing the health of elderly people

Introduction

In England and Wales about 140,000 hospital beds are occupied by people over the age of 65 years and a further 155,000 people are living in hostels or other institutions (3, 9). Thus about 4·6 per cent of the elderly population ($6·4 \times 10^6$ over 65 years) are resident in institutions at any one time, many permanently.

Many of these patients have degenerative conditions, such as osteo-arthritis, cardiovascular and cerebrovascular disorders, and dementias. Admission may be precipitated by an initial episode, such as a stroke, but many of these disorders develop insidiously. In these cases, entry to an institution, or entry to the waiting-list, may result from acute episodes of sickness which may or may not be directly related to the chronic process. In the presence of a chronic disability, and perhaps a long-standing strain upon relatives, any acute setback and its aftermath may disturb a precarious social adaptation in a manner which is difficult to reverse. Sickness in relatives may have the same effect, as may other transient or persisting disturbances in the social environment of the patient. With increasing age a progressively greater proportion of elderly people migrate into institutions of various kinds from which movement back into the community, or movement where necessary into a more appropriate institution, becomes increasingly difficult. Those remaining in the community are progressively 'selected' on the basis of their relative fitness to do so, both social and medical.

A great part of the medical care task in the elderly hinges upon the maintenance of fitness in this combined sense, and depends jointly upon (i) the level of social competence and adaptation and (ii) the presence or absence of life-threatening or disabling illness.

Adaptation to the community can be destroyed by an overwhelming setback in either field and there may be little that can be done. However, failures can occur because of moderate setbacks, or even quite minor setbacks if they occur in both fields together. This is where timely assistance can be most valuable.

Many surveys of elderly persons living in the community have been carried out in order to identify unsuspected pathologies (2, 8, 13) and others have investigated the take-up of social services (1). However, few have set out to make a joint medical/social assessment in functional terms, and to inquire into the feasibility of maintaining social fitness through surveillance and timely assistance. This is the purpose of a programme of work of which this report is a part. It is based upon a randomized trial of surveillance procedures carried out in a group of elderly people living in Harborne, a suburb of Birmingham. The needs of this group are to be monitored over a period of time and the effects of regular surveillance measured. At the same time the logistic and staffing problems of maintaining an adequate level of surveillance are to be examined. It is this last aspect which forms the basis of the present report and the results constitute, in effect, an exploration of the role of nurses in maintaining fitness in elderly people.

MATERIALS AND METHODS

The investigation was conducted in a general practice staffed by five doctors. Four district nurses and two health visitors were 'attached' by arrangement with the area health authority. An additional research nurse was seconded to the practice from the health services research centre for the purposes of the experiment and, as well as undertaking many of the visits, she has been responsible for the day-to-day running of the experiment. About 13,000 persons are registered with the practice and almost all live within five miles of the purpose-built group practice premises.

An experimental computer-based information system, designed for purposes of research, service-scheduling, and practice-activity analysis, has been in operation in the practice for the past three years (6). This system formed the basis for selecting and identifying a random sample of elderly persons. Approximately 8 per cent (1,040) of the people registered with the practice were over the age of 70 years. Not all were living at home. A one-in-eight sample of those people who were in fact living at home was selected and where other elderly persons registered with the same practice were found to be living in selected households, they were added to the 'study' group. The study group therefore amounted to 15 per cent of all the elderly persons.

Each nurse was allocated a number of patients in a limited geographical area. At the initial visit a structured social history was obtained and recorded on a questionnaire form, the recent usage of medical services was documented, an assessment of physical performance was made, and blood was taken for a biochemical profile.

Results

The findings are presented under five main headings related to (1) accessibility, (2) social circumstances, (3) patterns of service provision and usage, (4) medical and socio-medical problems, (5) logistics of surveillance.

ACCESSIBILITY

Ten of the 136 persons in the random sample were found to be dead, 7·4 per cent. The interval between their deaths and the visit by the nurse varied between two weeks and twenty years. It is easy to understand the continued inclusion on a GP's list of a patient who has recently died, but only six of the ten cases could be accounted for in this way. The longer-term failures of the information system had occurred despite the fact that the whole of the Executive Council list had in this case been copied, validated through a computer process, checked manually against the practice list and a large number of errors and inconsistencies reconciled (7). These findings do not appear to be isolated and the problem has been shown to exist in other areas (11).

Another 11 of the 136 had moved from the district but were still on the practice list. Thus, the deaths and migrations together resulted in some 15·4 per cent of initial visits failing to find a subject.

The majority of persons visited welcomed the nurse, but six refused interview and six were otherwise not available: some at work. This brings the total failed-contact rate to 22·2 per cent of the initial sample, or 10·4 per cent of those living and still available in the district. Altogether, 127 patients were interviewed, comprising 103 from the random sample, together with 24 found to be living in the same house and registered with the same practice. Before departing the nurse asked if she could visit again and in almost all cases this was welcomed. A second round of visits was planned for eight weeks later and this has since been completed. Altogether 122 patients, 96 per cent of the 127 interviewed on the first occasion, have been successfully visited again.

Although access was obtained to the majority of those approached, not all initial visits were completed without some difficulty. In the early part of the survey patients were asked if they would take part in a 'research project'. In practice this was not very acceptable and caused some apprehension and, apart from the six people who refused to be interviewed, some contacted the GP after the nurse had left, to confirm her authority and intentions. Following this experience the initial introduction was changed to one with a more personal approach in which it was explained that the doctor had asked the nurse to call on patients over the age of 70 years to check that all was well. Following this there were no further refusals and fewer patients sought confirmation from the practice.

There was also some difficulty with some of the procedures. Although all 127 subjects reacted favourably to pulse and blood pressure recording, two refused venepuncture and one refused a urine sample. In addition the nurses were unable to draw sufficient blood from 12 patients and 17 patients were unable to provide urine specimens.

SOCIAL CIRCUMSTANCES

Half the patients interviewed in the original sample were living alone, one-third were living with their husband or wife, and almost all the remainder were living with other relatives. Details are given in Table 1. A smaller proportion of men than women were living alone, and because men constituted only one-third of the sample, the absolute number of men living alone (8) was very much less than the number of women (45). This is partly due to differential mortalities in males and females, but may also possibly result from selective removal of men living alone from the community into institutional care or into the homes of relatives.

One curious feature of Table 1 deserves comment; it appears that more men are living with their wives than women are living with their husbands. At first sight this seems impossible, but several explanations can be advanced. First, there might be an effect of sampling variation. Second it is possible that elderly men living alone are removed preferentially from the community, into institutions. Third, it might be due to differences in the relative ages of wives and husbands; that is, our age-based sample has preferentially selected elderly males with surviving non-elderly wives as opposed to elderly females, many of whose older husbands have already died.

Almost all the elderly people in the sample catered for themselves but friends and relatives provided meals in eight cases, and the meals-on-wheels services in three, together amounting to 8·7 per cent of the total group interviewed.

TABLE 1

Living arrangements

	Living alone	Living with spouse	Living with other relatives but not spouse	Living with non-relatives	Total
Males	8	20 (3)	3	0	31
Females	45	11 (2)	14	2	72
Total	53	31	17	2	103

Figures in parenthesis denote those subjects living with other relatives as well as their spouse.

This table does not include the 24 persons subsequently added to the original sample of 103.

Each patient was classified on a five-point mobility scale, ranging from 'totally ambulant' through 'ambulant but housebound', 'semi-ambulant' (that is needing assistance), 'bedfast or chairfast' (but not totally helpless), to 'totally helpless'. The majority of subjects, 76 per cent, were 'totally ambulant', and none was 'totally helpless'. Twenty-one patients (16·5 per cent) were 'ambulant but housebound', 8 (6·5 per cent) were 'semi-ambulant', and 2 (1·6 per cent) were 'bedfast or chairfast'. The living conditions of the 26 per cent who were less than totally ambulant are particularly important from the point of view of maintaining their adaptation to community living. Of the 31 persons in this group (12 men and 19 women), 7 were living alone.

Most of the elderly people in the sample received reasonably frequent visits from friends and relatives, but many did not. Eleven patients had not had any visitors during the week preceding the visit and another 22 had received only one visitor during this week. These two groups together amount to 26 per cent of all persons interviewed. These data also relate importantly to living arrangements; of the 53 persons living alone, 25 per cent had received not more than one visitor in the previous week. Only 10 patients had received a professional visitor in the previous week, and even with a regular medical/nursing surveillance system in operation it would be a mistake to conclude that a realistic relief from loneliness would be provided in this way.

THE PROVISION AND USAGE OF THE HEALTH SERVICES

Almost three-quarters of the patients (74 per cent), with equal proportions of males and females, had consulted their practitioner during the preceding twelve months, but 8 per cent of the sample had not consulted their doctor for more than five years. A full distribution is given in Table 2.

TABLE 2

Interval between the last consultation with the GP and the nurse's visit

	0–6 weeks	6 weeks– 6 months	6 months– 1 year	1–5 years	More than 5 years	Total
Male	14 (37)	8 (21)	6 (16)	5 (13)	5 (13)	38 (100)
Female	26 (29)	26 (29)	14 (16)	18 (20)	5 (6)	89 (100)
Total	40 (31)	34 (27)	20 (16)	23 (18)	10 (8)	127 (100)

Figures in parenthesis are percentages.

The patients were asked whether they had been admitted to hospital during the preceding twelve months and whether they were having regular hospital out-patient appointments. Four of the males (10 per cent) and 5 of the females (6 per cent) had been in-patients; 3 of these admissions had been for ophthalmic treatment, 4 for other surgery. Equal proportions of males and females (20 per cent of each) had regular out-patient appointments. Ten of the 25 attendances were for ophthalmic conditions, the remainder covering a wide range of medical problems.

Tables 3 and 4 show the relationship between attendance at hospital and consultation with the GP. No patient was admitted to hospital without also seeing his GP during the year, and only two attended out-patients without having GP consultations. There is therefore no evidence that attendance was used as a substitute for primary consultation with a GP.

A record was made of the types and quantities of drugs that each subject was taking regularly; 22 males (57 per cent) and 42 females (47 per cent) were taking regular medication. The most common groups of drugs prescribed were psychotropics (18 per cent of men and 20 per cent of women), and cardiovascular drugs including

hypotensives, diuretics, potassium supplements, and cardiac glycer-
ides (in 26 per cent of men and 28 per cent of women). Twenty-five
per cent of patients were receiving medication for more than one
condition. Fourteen patients receiving cardiovascular and/or psycho-
tropic drugs had not consulted their GP for more than six months.

TABLE 3

Relationship between out-patient appointments and GP consultations

	Seen in last year by GP	Not seen in last year by GP	Total
Out-patient visits in last year	19 (15)	2 (2)	21 (17)
No out-patient visits	75 (59)	31 (24)	106 (83)
Total	94 (74)	33 (26)	127 (100)

Note. Total number of out-patient appointments 25, ie 4
patients have appointments at 2 clinics.
Figures in parenthesis are percentages.

TABLE 4

Relationship between hospital admission and GP consultations

	Seen in last year by GP	Not seen in last year by GP	Total
Admitted to hospital in last year	9 (7)	0	9 (7)
No hospital admission in last year	85 (67)	33 (26)	118 (93)
Total	94 (74)	33 (26)	127 (100)

Figures in parenthesis are percentages.

MEDICAL AND SOCIOMEDICAL PROBLEMS

As a result of the first visit, 14 patients (11 per cent) were referred to
their doctors. Three of the 14 were referred for immediate review of
their conditions, including two patients with dementias who were not
taking their drugs correctly, and a patient with chronic bronchitis
who had become chairfast and had developed a large inguinal hernia.
Two patients were referred with a view to the provision of hearing
aids and a further 2 for ear syringing. Seven patients presented with
new diagnoses including heart disease, hypertension, depression and
paranoia, lymphoedema, otitis externa, aplastic anaemia (diagnosed

after investigations in hospital) and a case of vaginal atrophy following a repair seven years ago about which the patient had been too embarrassed to consult her doctor; she has now been referred for gynaecological opinion.

Blood pressures were distributed as shown in Table 5; one man and five women had systolic readings of 200 mmHg or above, and one man and ten women had diastolic readings over 100 mmHg.

TABLE 5

The distribution of systolic and diastolic blood pressures

	mmHg							
	60–75	*80–95*	*100–15*	*120–45*	*150–95*	*200+*	*NK*	*Total*
Systolic pressure	0	0	7	41	72	6	1	127
Diastolic pressure	19	77	28	2	0	0	1	127

Only one of the patients was already receiving treatment; and only one was referred for treatment because she had symptoms. The others are remaining for the time being under surveillance without treatment.

The mean weight of the men was 69·5 kg (153 lb) and of the women 56·0 kg (123 lb). Three men and six women weighed more than 80 kg (176 lb), the heaviest weighing 95 kg (209 lb). None was seriously disabled from obesity alone, but several suffered from other chronic ailments such as congestive heart failure or osteo-arthritis and their obesity must put at risk their continued adaptation to the community. None of them has yet been referred for treatment specifically because they are overweight. Two women weighed less than 40 kg (88 lb) and the lightest man weighed 45 kg (99 lb). No specific nutritional deficiencies were noted.

Venous blood samples were taken from 113 subjects and the following serum estimations were made: urea, creatinine, uric acid, calcium, albumen, globulin, total bilirubin, alkaline phosphatase, SGOT, and cholesterol. Many patients displayed deviations of one or more values and 9 were found to have sufficiently abnormal results to warrant further investigation. Details of the 9 patients are given in Table 6. Two showed elevated alkaline phosphatase, 2 showed raised levels of serum urea, creatinine, and uric acid, 2 showed elevated serum urea with no other evidence of renal disease; the others showed a variety of excess values. Four months after the first visit none of these problems has been resolved any further. We

TABLE 6

The significantly abnormal biochemical results found in the sample

Patients	Urea mg/100 ml	Creatinine mg/100 ml	Uric acid mg/100 ml	Globulin g/100 ml	Total bilirubin mg/100 ml	Alkaline phosphatase K-a-units/100ml	SGOT IU/L	Cholesterol mg/100 ml
1	72							
2					4·1		63	
3	62							
4	49			3·9				324
5						85·0		
6	61	1·8	10·0					
7	48	1·8	9·2					
8						14·0		
9								113

suspect that 2 patients have chronic renal disease but have no explanation for the abnormal findings in the others. None of the patients has received any treatment or modification of treatment as a result of the blood examination.

In addition to the medical problems described above, the first visit revealed a number of social problems. As a result, 13 cases were referred to the Social Services departments to obtain 'home help', chiropody, or loans of equipment, or to the Birmingham Council for Old People, or for additional home nursing. Only four of these patients were referred for chiropody but the number might have been larger if the available resource had been greater.

Among the social and medical problems unveiled were a number of complex cases presenting several simultaneous problems. These are exemplified by one overweight chronic bronchitic who was blind and completely chairfast and whose wife had been struggling alone to cope with a difficult home situation. Like many similar situations it does not lend itself to any fully satisfactory resolution but a bath attendant was arranged, contact was re-established with the Welfare for the Blind Association, some social activities have been organized, and the family remains under surveillance.

Apart from the results of the biochemical screen and the further investigations arising from it, the first round of visits revealed 27 patients (21 per cent) for whom help was needed for either a medical or a social problem whose presence could be detected very simply by a nurse working to a scheduled plan of surveillance. In addition we must anticipate that a certain number of fresh problems will arise during the course of surveillance and that existing problems, not mentioned at the first visit, will be brought forward later. Indeed, the second visit, now complete, is confirming this supposition. Six more patients have been referred to their doctors, two for chest pains on exertion, one for increasingly frequent 'black-outs', one with gross distention of the abdomen, one with digitalis overdose, and one with loss of control of his previously known diabetes. In addition, five of the original referrals to the Social Services department have required repeat referral as no contact had been established and eight new cases have had to be referred.

LOGISTICS OF SURVEILLANCE

The basis of the surveillance programme was an up-to-date list of all people registered at the practice, characterized by age and sex. A comprehensive surveillance programme which does not depend upon the patient's spontaneous presentation cannot be undertaken at all unless such a register is available. In this case the register was prepared by computer although they can, of course, be prepared by hand. The 136 subjects in the random sample generated 187 nurse visits. Ninety-eight patients (72 per cent) were contacted or accounted for at the first visit; 25 (18 per cent) at the second; and 13 (10 per cent) at the third. This process resulted in 103 interviews. Each complete interview thus required approximately 1·8 visits, while the interview itself took between 40 and 45 minutes, as a rule. If a total population is covered, however, there will be some small savings in visiting time where two old people are living together. For example, our 103 successful visits in fact accessed 127 patients. In addition to the time taken on unfruitful visits a good deal of inquiry was required of neighbours when patients could not be contacted.

Experience of second visits suggests that the number of journeys necessary and the amount of time taken, for each successful interview, might be expected to decline. For resource projection purposes we might perhaps allow 1·5 journeys per interview over-all, and a mean interview time of 30 minutes. On this basis, the resource required for regular two-monthly visiting of every patient over 70 in the practice (13,000 patients altogether, with 1,040 over 70) would amount to 187 journeys per week and 62 hours of interview time.

A more general formula might be $n \times$ (24 journeys $+$ 8 hours interview) per week, for 10,000 total population, where $n =$ the number of interviews planned each year for each patient. In practical terms and depending on local circumstances, one visitor might be responsible for a total population of 25,000, spending the whole of her time in visiting over-70s on a once-a-year basis. On a five-times-a-year basis, a single visitor could cope with the geriatric surveillance problems arising in a total population of about 5,000 persons, that is about 400 elderly people.

Discussion

Although this is a small-scale project and needs to be repeated in different populations and in different practices, six reasonably precise conclusions can be drawn.

1. A first conclusion is that the investigation has revealed a clear need for unsolicited visiting of elderly people living at home. This is true whether the need is measured in terms of unreported problems detected, or whether it is assessed in the more stringent terms of those amenable to assistance. In addition, although it was not encountered in this small survey, there is the general problem of the neglected recluse who never presents volitionally to medical or social services. Follow-up revealed that a substantial secondary yield of problems appears at a second visit and it is likely that new problems will continue to be revealed at later visits still, although probably at lower frequencies than at the first two.

2. A second conclusion is that this important group of problems is within the capacity of a nurse to detect. Much of it is a matter of asking very simple questions and making very simple observations. This conclusion is supported by McNabola (10). Only a limited clinical examination is called for and much of its value (for example, of taking the blood pressure and weight) is to establish an apparent concrete purpose for the visit and thus to assist in access. The urinary and blood examinations seem to be of quite doubtful marginal value, especially if they prolong the visit beyond the time which is economic within available resources or if they reduce the acceptability of visiting. These are questions which probably deserve repeated inquiry.

3. A third conclusion is that a considerable staff resource would be needed if every person over 70 were to be visited regularly at the frequency initially undertaken in this study, that is about six times per year. There are about 4×10^6 persons of 70 years or more in England and Wales (12), and a total of approximately 20,000 non-hospital nurses and health visitors, excluding midwives and pupil midwives (4). Not all of the latter are whole-time. If, as we calculate, a whole-time nurse can cope with the surveillance needs of about 400 elderly persons on a five-times-a-year basis, we would need to occupy more than half of the available non-hospital nursing and health-visitor work force entirely on this task. We do not appear to have any estimates of the equivalent work force *currently* employed on the care of elderly people, but it is almost certainly much less than this.

The 20,000 staff referred to above include only 6,000 health visitors, so the problem of meeting surveillance needs at the standard adopted in the study would be entirely hopeless if limited to them. This discrepancy was pointed out by Donald (5).

If regular surveillance of elderly people is to be contemplated as a national policy, it will require the abandonment of any procedures which prolong visits unnecessarily; and any procedures which require re-visiting at short intervals, or which reduce the acceptability of visiting to the patient. It is also clear that the surveillance task would have to be seen as a proper responsibility of all nursing-staff groups and not be limited either to home nurses or to health visitors. Finally, the mean frequency of repeat visits will probably have to be less than six per year and this would then necessitate either a limited primary selection of those requiring initial visiting, or some basis for varying the intervals between successive visits according to needs assessed at the first.

Research directed towards these ends obviously requires some immediate attention.

4. The fourth conclusion is that surveillance procedures must be based upon population lists. Most general practice record systems are not organized in such a manner as to permit the scheduling of regular checks which do not depend upon the initiatives of the patients themselves. We have found that even when a practice age/sex register was constructed a substantial proportion of initial attempts to contact patients failed. There is no reciprocal mechanism whereby failures related to other practices could be collected. A total population register must be available *somewhere* if a surveillance scheme such as this is to be completely successful; the re-attachment to general medical services of patients who have lost contact, must be one of the objectives of surveillance.

5. Another conclusion, or perhaps a question, relates to the optimal terms of attachment of nursing and health visitor staffs to GPs. A surveillance programme cannot depend upon spontaneous demands for GP services, but in large part precedes and even generates those demands. Furthermore, as we have seen, the organization of a surveillance service will require an independently designed information system. Attachment schemes confer benefits to both nurses and doctors through mutual contact and education, and on patients through providing secondary nursing services following traditional 'on-demand' GP contacts; in addition part at least of a surveillance programme, for example relating to the proper administration of drugs, can be initiated from such contacts. Indeed, they form a part-basis for the selective requirements mentioned above. Likewise, the process of referring patients found to be in need is assisted by the personal and joint working contacts established in an attachment scheme. However, the findings of this study indicate that attachment schemes must be seen as part of, and not a substitute for, a global responsibility for the total elderly population of a geographically defined area, for example an administrative district or an administrative area of the NHS.

6. Finally (and again perhaps a question rather than a conclusion) our findings have implications relating to the optimal training and job descriptions of nursing staffs. The issue is partly a question of numbers and partly a question of the optimal employment of existing staff and the avoidance of duplicate visiting. There is a question whether nursing activities should continue to be based, as at present, on a division between home nurses and health visitors, or whether a more comprehensive and unified training and responsibility should be defined for this age-group and indeed for other age-groups too. It is likely, for example, that the issue could be stated in a very similar form in relation to child care and surveillance services. If surveillance services for children, elderly people, the handicapped, the mentally subnormal and the mentally sick, together with the screening services appropriate to middle life, come jointly to constitute a substantial part of our medical care programmes, some such solution will have to be devised.

Summary

A study of medical/social problems was carried out in a random sample of a general practice population. The initial investigation of these problems was carried out by nurses. A need for unsolicited visiting of the elderly was established and the suitability of nurses to carry out this task was confirmed. The logistics of visiting were investigated and it was discovered that present numbers of available nurses would not permit regular visiting of all elderly people to be adopted as a national policy.

There are immediate requirements for (1) research to devise bases for selective visiting, and (2) re-consideration of the tasks, training and job descriptions of nurses engaged on this work.

ACKNOWLEDGEMENTS
This study is part of an on-going programme of work related to the development of information systems in general practice. The programme of work is undertaken jointly by the Birmingham Health Services Research Centre and the Harborne Study Practice of the Royal College of General Practitioners (Professor E. G. Knox and Dr D. L. Crombie). Particular thanks for their participation in this part of the programme go to the nurses and health visitors who have taken part, Miss L. Bull, Mrs J. Hall, Mrs P. Jinks, Mrs J. Morgan, and Mrs F. Woods. Grateful thanks are also due to Dr P. Wilding of the Wolfson Research Laboratories and Dr R. D. T. Farmer of the Department of Community Medicine, Westminster Medical School, London.

References

1. COOPER, B. (1971). 'Social work in general practice—the Derby scheme', *Lancet*, **i**, 539–42.
2. CURRIE, G., MACNEILL, R. M., WALKER, J. G., BARNIE, E., and MUDIE, E. W. (1974). 'Medical and social screening of patients aged 70–72 by an urban general practice health team', *Br. med. J.* **2**, 108–11.
3. DHSS (1972). *Health—Personal Social Services Statistics* (London: HMSO).
4. —— (1973). *Health—Personal Social Services Statistics* (London: HMSO).
5. DONALD, A. G. (1971). 'Health visitor attachment', *Teach In*, **1**, 305.
6. FARMER, R. D. T. F., and CROSS, K. W. (1972). 'An automated records system for general practice', *Br. J. prev. soc. Med.* **26**, no. 3, 148–52.
7 —— KNOX, E. G., CROSS, K. W., and CROMBIE, D. L. (1974). 'Executive Council lists and general practitioner files', ibid. **28**, no. 1, 49–53.
8. HISCOCK, E., PRANGNELL, D. R., and WILMOT, J. F. (1973). 'A screening survey of old people in a general practice', *Practitioner*, **210**, 271–7.
9. KING'S HOSPITAL FUND CENTRE (1970). 'Care for the elderly' (Editorial), *Community Med.* no. 3302, **126**, no. 20, 266.
10. McNABOLA, E. K. A. (1970). 'An assessment of the elderly by a district nursing sister attached to a group practice', *Health Bull. (Edinb.)*, **28**, no. 1, 9–12.
11. MOORE, P. E., and CROSS, K. W. (1972). 'Preliminary survey of the needs of the elderly in Shrewsbury', *Community Med.* **128**, 101–3.
12. REGISTRAR GENERAL FOR ENGLAND AND WALES (1970). *Statistical Review* (London: HMSO).
13. WILLIAMS, E. I., BENNETT, F. M., NIXON, J. V., NICHOLSON, ROSANEL, and GABERT, J. (1972). 'Sociomedical study of patients over 75 in general practice', *Br. med. J.* **2**, 445–8.

T. Marshall
MSc
R. D. T. Farmer*
MBBS, MRCEP
K. W. Cross
BSc, PhD
Health Services Research Centre
Department of Social Medicine
University of Birmingham

*Now at the Department of Community
Medicine, Westminster Medical School,
London

A new method of comparing consulting patterns in general practice

A new method of comparing consulting patterns in general practice

Introduction

In many countries, including the United Kingdom, the GP is the main provider of primary medical care. He is directly accessible to the members of the community which he serves; he treats many ailments himself without reference to other medical services; and sometimes he refers patients to more specialist facilities for diagnosis and/or treatment. Numerically, the GP often dominates a health care system and he assumes a greater importance by his ability to consume other resources on behalf of his patients. For these reasons it is important to understand the dynamics of general practice utilization by populations and by subgroups of populations. A prerequisite to such an undertaking is the development of suitable statistical summarizing indices which provide the maximum amount of information in a concise and intelligible form without the need for expensive and time-consuming data acquisition systems. An index should be sufficiently sensitive to allow comparison of demand and usage patterns in different groups of people according to age, sex, social class, diagnosis, or any other demographic or medical variable; and ideally it should assist in the formulation of particular practice management policies and be useful in the assessment of the effect of change.

INDICES IN COMMON USE AND THEIR DIFFICULTIES

Consulting rates and episode rates are the most common methods of summarizing practice utilization data. The episode rate is calculated by dividing the total number of *episodes* of illness in a given time, in a given population, by the size of that population. The result is then expressed in a time-dimensioned manner, that is x episodes of illness per 1,000 persons in unit time. The consulting rate is similarly calculated by dividing the total number of consultations by the size of the population.

These rates are easy to calculate but suffer from three major disadvantages: (1) lack of objectivity in the numerator; (2) the definition of the denominator; and (3) inherent difficulties in making statistical comparisons.

1. Objectivity of numerator

Because of the indefinite nature of its beginning and its end, an episode of illness can be difficult to define. Most investigators who have used this term attempt to circumvent the difficulty by counting each single diagnosis as an episode however often throughout the survey period the patient may consult for it. Thus, if a patient with a peptic ulcer consults his doctor on one or more occasions during a survey period it is counted as a single episode however far apart in time the consultations may have occurred. In effect, this makes the episode rate synonymous with 'new diagnosis rate'. Even in the formalized sense of 'new diagnosis rate', the episode rate lacks that objectivity which would make it suitable for comparative studies. Doctors behave differently in their use of provisional, definitive, and multiple diagnosis; for example, changes in diagnoses without changes in symptoms inflate the number of episodes and introduce ambiguity. In complex situations it is possible for there to be more 'episodes' than consultations. The episode rate is further complicated by the inclusion of episodes which begin before the survey period, yet continue to generate consultations within it. In cases such as this the time dimensionality is altered. Whilst the examination of episode rate provides interesting insights into the diagnostic idiosyncrasies of individual practitioners it cannot provide a reproduceable statistic for comparative studies.

In some cases it has been assumed that a constant relationship exists between the number of episodes and the number of consultations but, unless this can be demonstrated, the episode rate cannot be used as a consistent comparative criterion. We are not aware of any studies which demonstrate a consistency of this kind.

A *consultation rate* does not suffer from the same difficulties as an episode rate. A consultation is defined as a meeting between a doctor and a patient, irrespective of any previous or current attempt at diagnosis. Therefore, the consultation rate has an objectivity not possessed by the episode rate.

2. Definition of the denominator

The definition of a denominator is a problem common to the use of both episode and consulting rates. The denominator that is usually used is the size of the population 'at risk' of having an episode of illness or a consultation during the period of the survey. Commonly in the UK this is taken as the number of people registered with a particular practitioner. It is assumed that if a doctor has accepted legal responsibility for providing medical care to a number of people, they are all equally at risk to consult him or use his services in other ways. However, it has been shown that people may leave an area without de-registering with a GP and other people may move into an area and fail to register until they need to consult (3). Some of the people registered with a GP may be in long-stay hospital units or in welfare homes; they are unlikely to consult as alternative care is provided for them. In many studies using consultation and episode rates it has not been clear whether the denominator was defined as the number of people registered at the Executive Council (now the Family Practitioner Committee), or the number of people for whom the doctors themselves hold records; these two numbers are rarely the same.

An alternative denominator sometimes used is the number of people consulting during the period of the investigation. The advantage of this denominator is that when a person consults he declares both his existence and the fact that he is at risk to that particular practitioner. Even so, it is possible for a person to consult at the beginning of a survey and leave before its end, or to consult only at the end of the survey having just moved into the catchment area of the practitioner. If the number of persons consulting is used it is likely that the number of exposed-to-risk patient-years will be over-estimated.

Denominator problems such as these assume great importance where there is high population mobility and it is in high mobility areas that many of the problems of medical care arise. The use of attendance denominators may be unavoidable in some places (for example, outside the UK) where GPs do not have defined 'lists' and it is then essential to declare the details of the computation and so avoid invoking false comparisons with episode or consultation rates calculated on other bases. Ideally a statistic summarizing utilization patterns should be denominator independent if it is to be used for comparative purposes.

3. Problems of statistical comparison

A consultation rate, or an episode rate, is in effect the arithmetic mean of the distribution of numbers of consultations or episodes in a population in unit time, and the form of the distribution presents problems of mathematical description and statistical comparisons. Over a limited period of time the distribution is characteristically non-modal and strongly skewed (Fig. 1). Because of this a given value of a single parameter (mean, or rate) can represent a range of widely different patterns. The mean takes account of persons nominally registered with a practitioner who do not consult, ie non-users. The wide variation in consultation rates may be explained by the denominator being incorrect, thus creating a spurious excess of non-users. Standard deviations of non-modal distributions have very limited meaning, and standard errors of means computed from this type of distribution do not supply a valid basis for assessing the significance of any differences that are detected.

Curve fitting techniques

A more sophisticated analysis of consultations in general practice was carried out by Froggatt *et al*. (4). They obtained the distribution of surgery attendances for 2,810 female patients continually registered with a three-doctor practice in Belfast during a three-year period, and tested four hypotheses by curve-fitting and correlation techniques for their respective abilities to explain the data. The data were found to be compatible with a 'proneness' hypothesis,[1] ie there was a good fit of a negative binomial distribution to the observed data; but this distribution did not fit the corresponding results for home visits. Froggatt *et al*. did not examine data for age/sex groups; however, Spencer (7) examined the Exeter survey data and found that, when combined into five age-groups, the data 'approximated particularly well' to the negative binomial distribution.

More recently Ashford (2) analysed the Exeter data collected during 1966–7 using five-year age-groups for all patient contacts including those who joined or left the practice during the survey. He found that the negative binomial distribution did not provide an adequate fit to all sets of data: for surgery attendances, agreement

---

1. 'Proneness' is a concept which implies that some people are more likely to attend *ab initio* than others, and that early attendance in a series tends to generate later attendances.

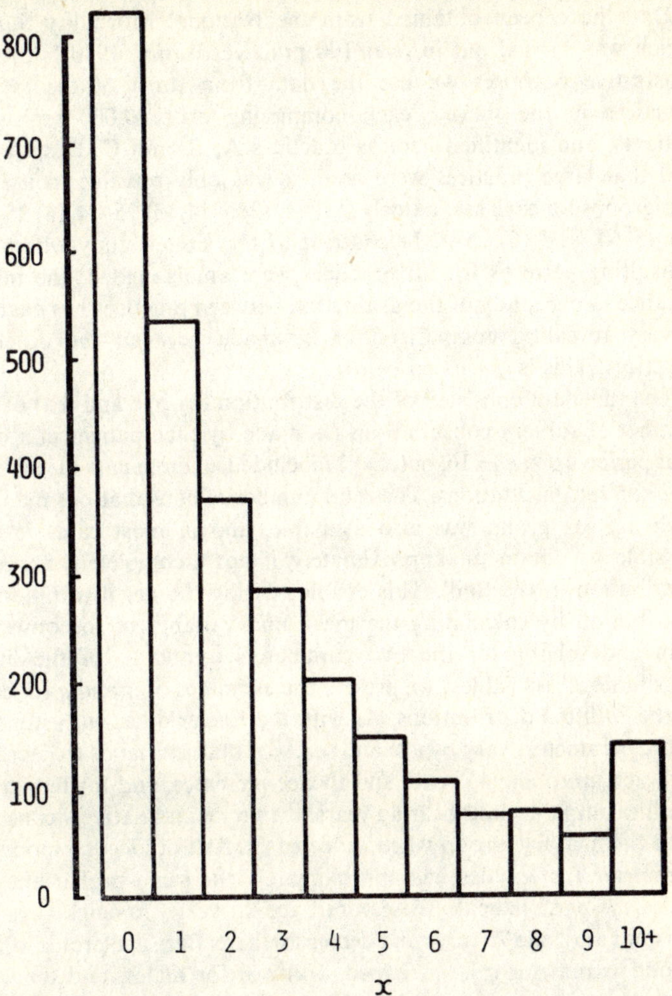

Figure 1. Distribution of the number of patients consulting x times during a year.

was particularly poor for males in the youngest age-groups and for females of all ages; for home visits the fit was better, although large discrepancies remained for females in the child-bearing age-groups, and above 75 years of age. In view of this conflicting evidence it seemed worthwhile to examine the applicability of the negative binomial distribution to other sets of data.

Data have been obtained from the National Morbidity Survey which was carried out in over 100 practices during 1970/1 (5); for illustrative purposes we use the data from three of the largest practices in the survey, each comprising over 10,000 registered patients, and identified here as practices **A**, **B**, and **C**. Despite the fact that large practices were used, it was only possible to use six age-groups for each sex, namely (1) 0–4, (2) 5–14, (3) 15–24, (4) 25–44, (5) 45–64, and (6) 65+. In contrast to the Exeter study where the consulting patterns for all practices were amalgamated, the maintenance in our study of the distinction between practices has enabled a very revealing comparison to be made between the different practices. This is discussed below.

The raw data consisted of the distribution (by age and sex) of the number of surgery consultations (x) made by each patient in a one-year period up to $x = 16$, but $x = 17$ included all those patients making 17 *or more* consultations. The total number of consultations made in each age/sex group was also available, and in most cases it was possible to obtain an approximately, if not a completely, accurate distribution in the 'tail'. This enabled fitting the negative binomial distribution by calculating the mean and variance of the observed data and solving for the two parameters w and q, of the fitted distribution.[1] In Table 1 we present the estimates of w and q for each of the 28 fitted distributions. As with the Exeter data, our estimates of the parameters vary by age and sex. For males, w tends to decrease with age up to age 45 years and thence increases, and for females it declines until the child-bearing years, then remains relatively constant until the final age-group when it decreases. Ashford's corresponding parameter for females has approximately the same profile but for males the parameter decreases until age 25 years, remains virtually constant until age 75 years and decreases thereafter. The profile of our second parameter q is U-shaped with age for males, and tends to increase with age for females; this parameter is not directly comparable with Ashford's second parameter. However, our prime concern is whether the parameters generate distributions which fit the observed data.

---

1. The probability density function of a random variable x which follows a negative binomial distribution is given by

$$f(x) = \binom{x+w-1}{x} p^{w} q^{x} \qquad \begin{array}{l} x = 0, 1, 2 \ldots \\ p+q = 1 \end{array}$$

with mean wq/p and variance wq/p^{2}. These are solved to give estimates of w, p, and q.

The goodness of fit of the negative binomial to the observed distributions was examined by χ^2 tests; the values of χ^2 are also given in Table 1 (cells were amalgamated so that no expected frequencies were less than 4), along with the probability level for the appropriate degrees of freedom (final number of cells minus 3). As in the Exeter study, most of the theoretical distributions were a good fit for the

TABLE 1

Parameter estimates and fits for the negative binomial distribution

Practice	Age-group	w	q	χ^2	df	Probability
Males						
A	1	1·26	0·71	9·85	11	$0\cdot5 < P < 0\cdot75$
C	1	1·16	0·74	13·39	10	$0\cdot1 < P < 0\cdot25$
A	2	0·72	0·70	6·15	10	$0\cdot75 < P < 0\cdot9$
B	2	0·97	0·68	8·36	12	$0\cdot75 < P < 0\cdot9$
C	2	0·90	0·64	11·09	8	$0\cdot1 < P < 0\cdot25$
A	3	0·69	0·65	15·72	7	$0\cdot025 < P < 0\cdot05$
B	3	0·89	0·66	10·67	9	$0\cdot25 < P < 0\cdot5$
C	3	0·78	0·64	9·83	7	$0\cdot1 < P < 0\cdot25$
A	4	0·55	0·72	20·50	10	$P = 0\cdot025$
C	4	0·49	0·75	8·42	11	$0\cdot5 < P < 0\cdot75$
A	5	0·66	0·79	16·14	12	$0\cdot1 < P < 0\cdot25$
C	5	0·67	0·78	10·58	13	$0\cdot5 < P < 0\cdot75$
A	6	0·79	0·82	8·64	12	$0\cdot5 < P < 0\cdot75$
B	6	1·02	0·81	21·86	10	$0\cdot01 < P < 0\cdot025$
C	6	0·64	0·78	22·32	11	$0\cdot01 < P < 0\cdot025$
Females						
A	1	1·19	0·69	12·90	10	$0\cdot1 < P < 0\cdot25$
B	1	1·63	0·68	13·76	11	$0\cdot1 < P < 0\cdot25$
A	2	0·74	0·69	8·81	10	$0\cdot5 < P < 0\cdot75$
B	2	0·99	0·70	6·71	12	$0\cdot75 < P < 0\cdot9$
C	2	0·97	0·62	15·58	7	$0\cdot025 < P < 0\cdot05$
A	3	0·78	0·79	27·23	13	$0\cdot01 < P < 0\cdot025$
C	3	0·75	0·77	22·47	12	$0\cdot025 < P < 0\cdot05$
A	4	0·80	0·77	38·95	13	$P < 0\cdot005$
C	4	0·78	0·79	34·64	13	$P < 0\cdot005$
A	5	0·69	0·79	25·84	13	$0\cdot01 < P < 0\cdot025$
C	5	0·91	0·74	62·85	13	$P < 0\cdot005$
B	6	0·76	0·83	25·85	11	$0\cdot005 < P < 0\cdot01$
C	6	0·51	0·81	22·25	13	$0\cdot01 < P < 0\cdot025$

males (11 out of 15 in our case), but the fit for female consultation data was satisfactory in only 4 out of 13 cases, and none of the four were in age-groups 15–24 or above. This again accords roughly with the Exeter study, and was interpreted as (in part) due to the effects of consultations for pregnancy, which could not be held to follow the same 'proneness' type of behaviour. (Such an explanation obviously cannot be used to explain the non-fit of consultation data of women above child-bearing age.) The more recent Exeter study (2) based upon episodes could perhaps be used to overcome this particular difficulty. However, for reasons given in the introduction we feel that episode rates are anyway unsatisfactory. Furthermore, as the authors themselves admitted in their reply to the discussion of their paper, their mathematically sophisticated approach is unlikely to be widely applied by managers in the health service.

A new approach

The fact that a number of studies have shown the negative binomial to be, sometimes, an appropriate functional form is useful in that it accords with the proneness hypothesis, and is consistent with that explanation of why patients consult their GPs. However, even when the negative binomial does fit, estimating the parameters q and w is not a trivial matter, and it is certainly something unlikely to be indulged in by any but the most numerate of GPs. As a simple tool for use by managers or by doctors themselves in describing patterns of consultation in general practice, the negative binomial cannot be accepted.

A simpler approach can be obtained by transforming the data of the frequency distribution to which the negative binomial is fitted. Instead of dealing with the number (or proportion) of patients making x consultations during a year, we use the number (proportion) making *at least r* consultations during the year (provided $r \geqslant 1$). When the negative binomial is appropriate, the algebraic form of the transformation is given in the appendix; verbally, the first point of the transformed data comprises the total number (or proportion) of patients consulting at all, the second point the total number (proportion) returning for a second consultation, the third point all those returning for a third consultation, and so on.

A typical example of the result of such a transformation is shown in Fig. 2, which looks rather like the histogram of a geometric progression with a common ratio less than 1. To examine this more closely, we required a set of data large enough to be unaffected (at least, grossly so) by the random fluctuations to be expected from small numbers in the tail of the distribution. Our own data, being

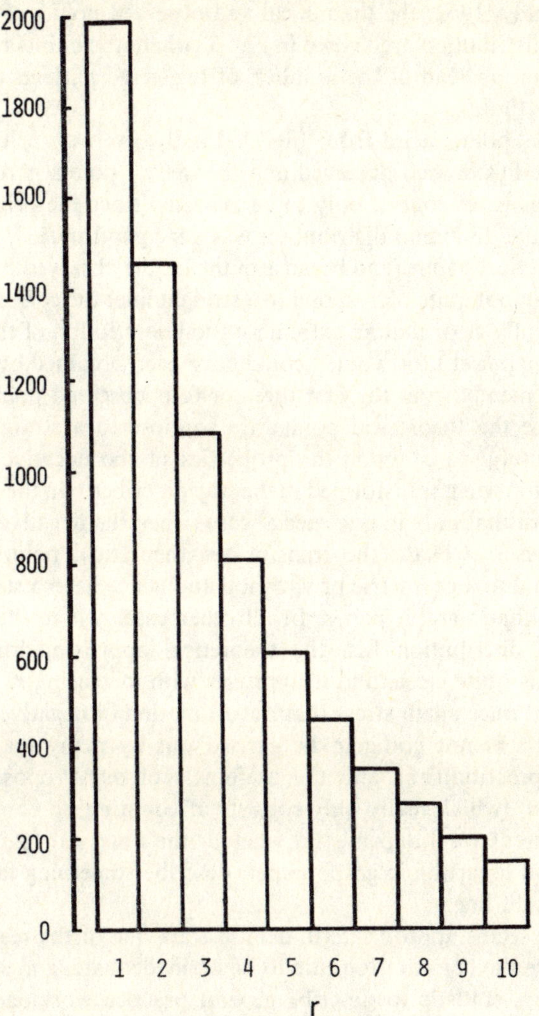

Figure 2. Distribution of the number of patients consulting at least *r* times during a year.

subdivided by both age and sex, was perhaps inadequate in this respect without amalgamation, but from Froggatt *et al.* (4) it was possible to obtain both theoretical and observed points for a far larger number of people (2,810 women) for one of the three years under study, 1962; the theoretical and observed points of the transformed distribution are shown in Fig. 3 (where the points refer to the proportion, instead of the number, of registered patients consulting at least r times).

Various points arise from Fig. 3. Firstly, even on a logarithmic scale, the fit between observed and theoretical points is remarkably good; this is, of course, only to be expected since the original fit of the negative binomial distribution was very good indeed. Secondly, the theoretical points (and because of the fit, the observed points too), almost but not quite correspond to a straight line; the correspondence is sufficiently close that an extremely good description of the over-all consulting pattern for women could have been obtained by an extrapolation merely from the first three or four observed points.

Because the theoretical points are so close to a straight line, it seemed useful to examine the properties of the negative binomial distribution when transformed in the way described. In the Appendix it is shown that only in one special case (when the negative binomial parameter $w = 1$) do the transformed theoretical points actually correspond to a geometric progression and hence lie in a straight line on logarithmic graph paper. In all other cases where the negative binomial distribution fits, the theoretical approximation to log-linearity is quite close, and it improves with increasing r. However, we should once again stress that the estimation of negative binomial parameters is not going to be carried out by many managers or general practitioners; and the usefulness of our proposed 'transformation' (which really only consists of counting up consultations in a different way) depends on whether the observed figures, when plotted on logarithmic graph paper, describe something fairly close to a straight line.

It now seems appropriate to demonstrate one of the reasons why we believe the consultation rate to be an inadequate, and sometimes misleading, statistic to describe general practice workload; and at the same time to show how our method, whilst still extremely simple, can impart more information. In practice C the consultation rate for males aged 0–4 was 3·374, and in practice B for males aged 45–64 it was 3·382. In Fig. 4 the proportions of the registered population consulting at least once, twice, etc., are plotted; the patterns of consultation are clearly quite different, with a higher proportion of the younger age-group consulting initially, but tending to reconsult less frequently than the middle-aged. Both sets of points can (roughly) be

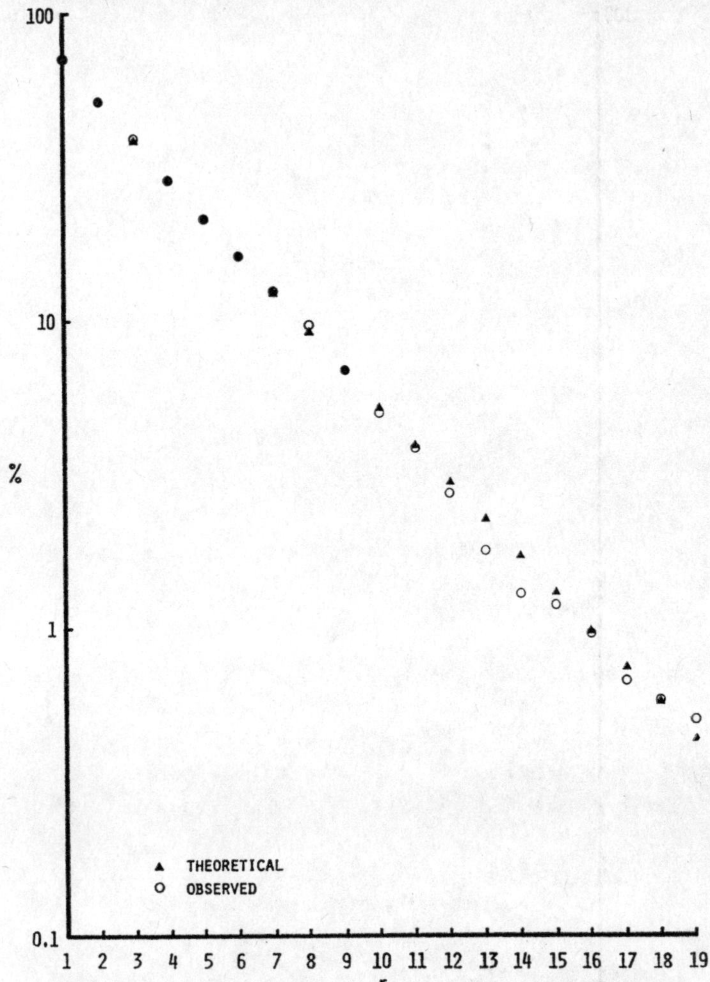

Figure 3. Proportion of patients consulting at least *r* times (from ref. 4).

characterized by an intercept (which corresponds to the proportion consulting) and a slope (which corresponds in some sense to a '*re*consultation rate'); and the intercepts and slopes for these two sets are obviously different, despite the fact that the over-all consultation rates are almost identical.

It is interesting to consider other types of contrast which can be

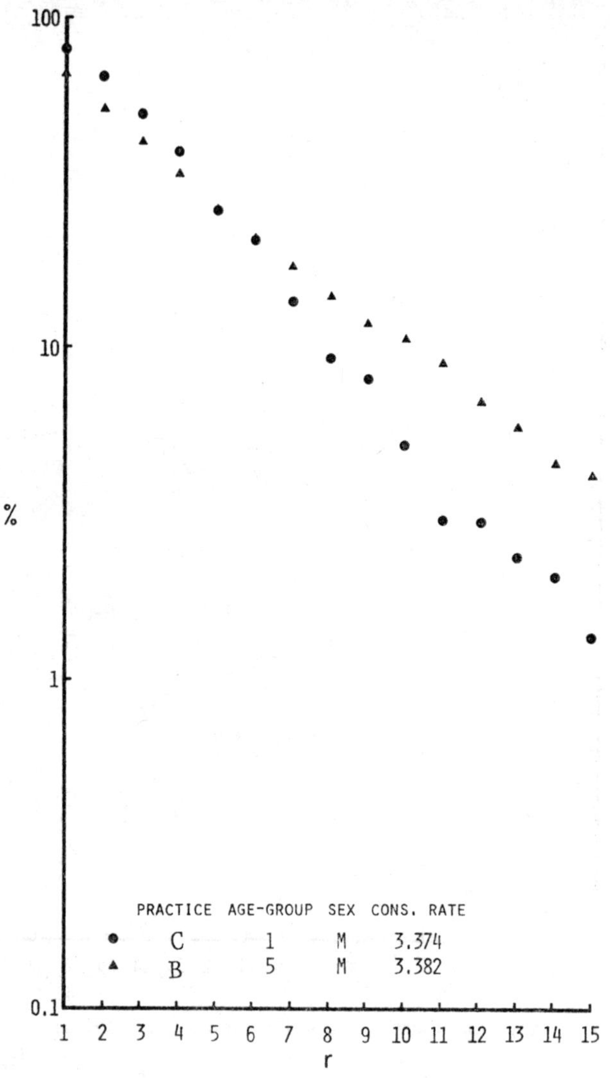

Figure 4. Observed proportion of patients consulting at least *r* times.

demonstrated by the plotting procedure. Fig. 5 shows the contrast between age-groups 1 and 2, ie between the 0–4 and 5–14 age-groups; more of the younger age-group consult than the older group, and they also consult more often. (Points approximately on a straight line

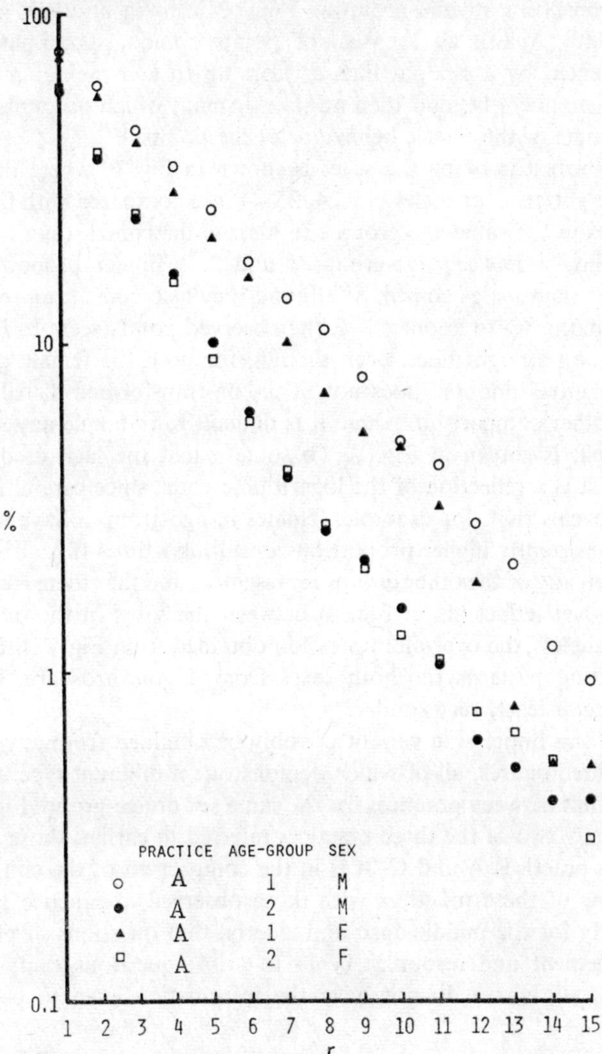

Figure 5. Observed proportion of patients consulting at least *r* times.

indicate a constant proportionate decline in the number (proportion) of patients making a further consultation; and parallel sets of points show the same proportionate decline between different groups, even through the absolute level from which they start, for example 80 per cent consulting in one group and 60 per cent in another, may be different.) Again, all the sets of points could approximately be represented by a straight line, at least up to and including $r = 8$; actual numbers beyond then are fairly small, which accounts for at least some of the erratic behaviour of the points.

A contrast between the sexes is shown in Fig. 6, where the consulting patterns for males (15–24, 25–44) are compared with those of females in the same age-groups. In a sense the contrast is similar to that shown between age-groups 1 and 2; a higher proportion of females than males consult at all, and they also consult more often. Once more, up to about $r = 8$ the observed points seem to lie very closely on straight lines, even though, for both the female groups, the negative binomial does not fit the un-transformed distribution.

Another comparison, where it is difficult to untangle any specific contrast, is shown in Fig. 7. To some extent the lack of obvious contrast is a reflection of the logarithmic scale, since careful inspection reveals that, for example, females in age-group 5 have a slight but consistently higher proportion consulting r times (for all r up to 13) than any of the other groups represented, and that there is a slight 'cross-over' effect (as in Fig. 4) between the sexes in the over-65s. Nevertheless, the over-all impression obtained from Fig. 7 is that the consulting patterns for both sexes from 45 onwards are, in this practice at least, very similar.

Such an impression cannot possibly be obtained from any of the next three figures, all of which demonstrate a different type of contrast, that between practices for the same sex or age-group. Figs. 5–7 used only two of the three practices referred to earlier, those identified as practices A and C. It is in the comparison of the consulting patterns of these practices with those observed in practice B, particularly for the middle-aged and elderly, that questions of practice management and resources begin to arise: questions that, in the present study, we do not have the information even to begin to answer.

Fig. 8 shows a comparison between practices A and B for both sexes in the 45–64 age-group. It is immediately clear (as it will be in the two subsequent diagrams) that a higher proportion of both males and females in practice B than in practice A are seen at all by their GP, and they are also seen more often. In addition (though this is not the main point) there is virtually no distinction between the consulting patterns of males and females in practice A, whereas in practice B

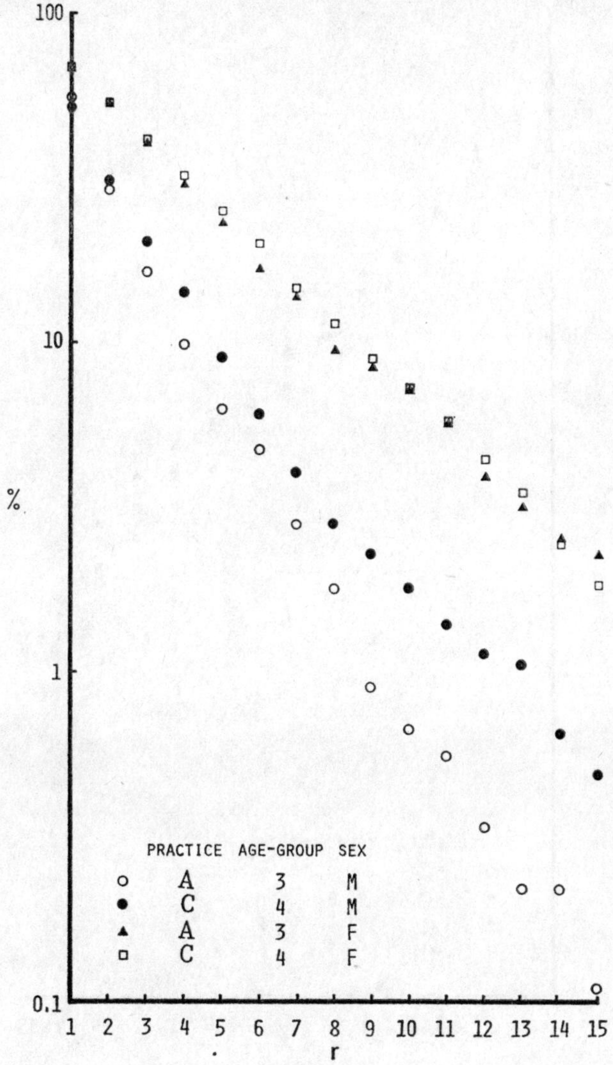

Figure 6. Observed proportion of patients consulting at least *r* times.

females are seen more often than males. Fig. 9 shows the contrast, for males alone this time, though for two age-groups, between practices B and C. Again in both age-groups a higher proportion of males consult their GP in practice B than in practice C and those that do

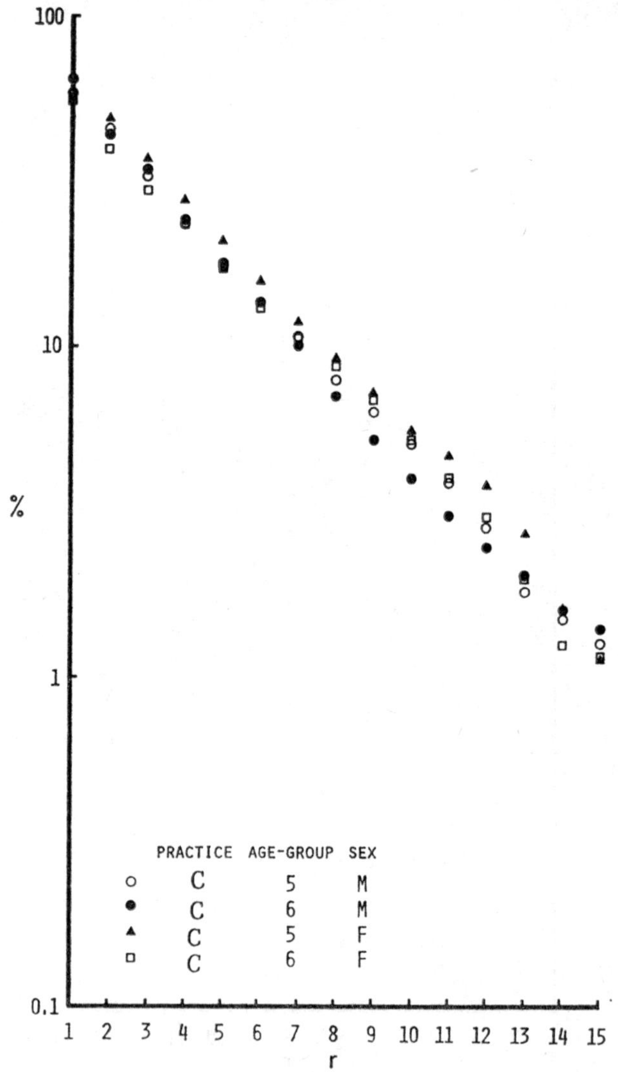

Figure 7. Observed proportion of patients consulting at least *r* times.

consult also consult more frequently. Apart from this contrast we should perhaps note that of all the consulting patterns so far seen, that of over-65 males in practice **B** is the one which diverges soonest (by $r = 6$) and remains most distinct, from a linear approximation.

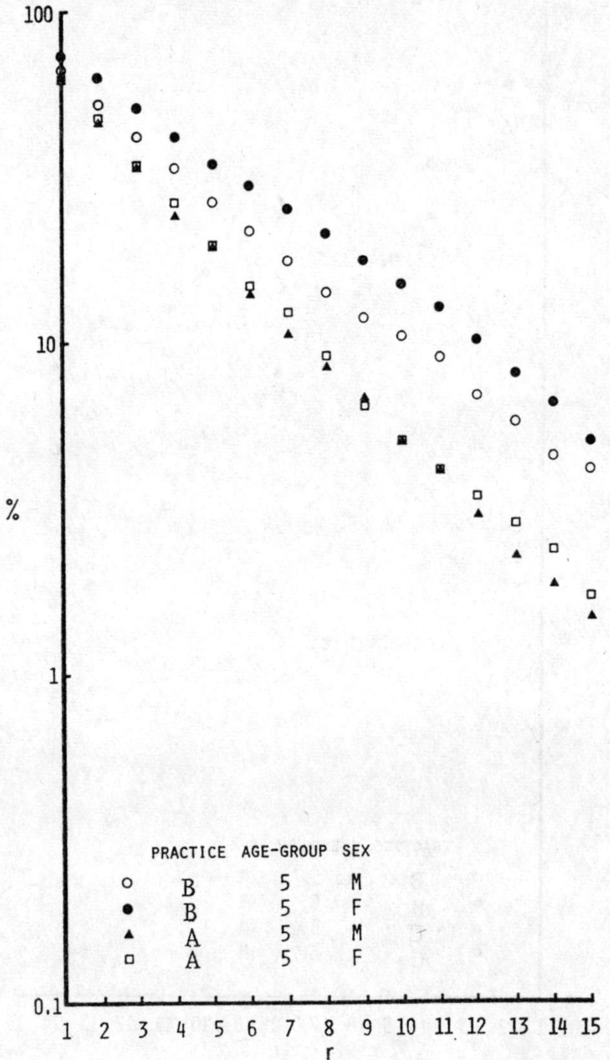

Figure 8. Observed proportion of patients consulting at least *r* times.

Finally, Fig. 10 shows the contrast between practices A and B for females only in two age-groups, 25–44 and 45–64. All four patterns approximate closely to linearity, the most divergent being the slight sigmoid shape of the consulting pattern for 45–64-year-old females

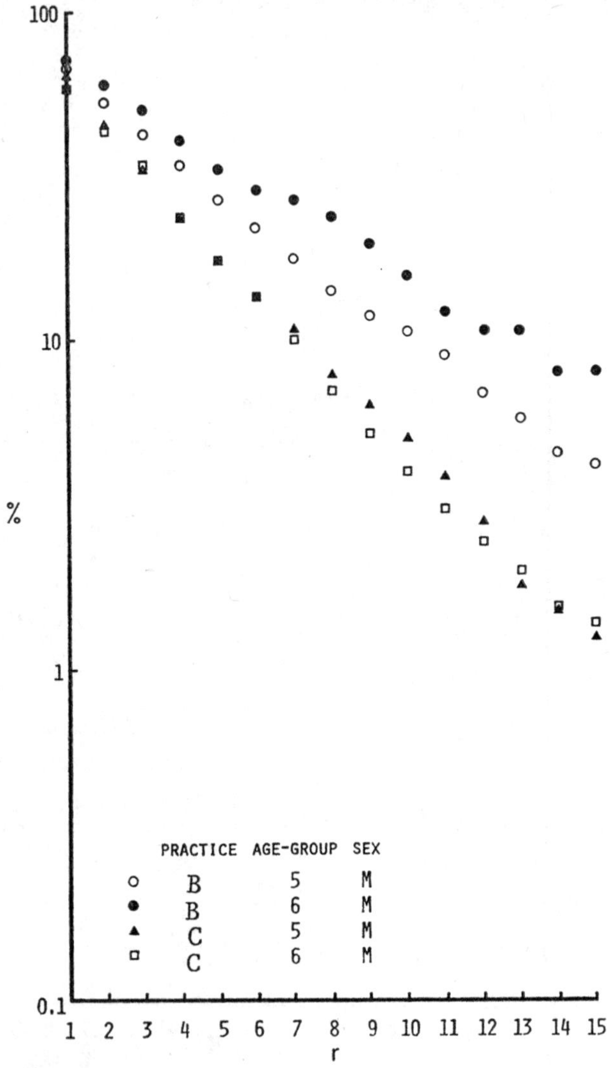

Figure 9. Observed proportion of patients consulting at least *r* times.

in practice B; this is perhaps more noticeable here than in Fig. 8 (where it also appeared) because it winds around another consulting pattern which is even closer to linearity.

It should be noted that in Figs. 5–10, we have covered all age and

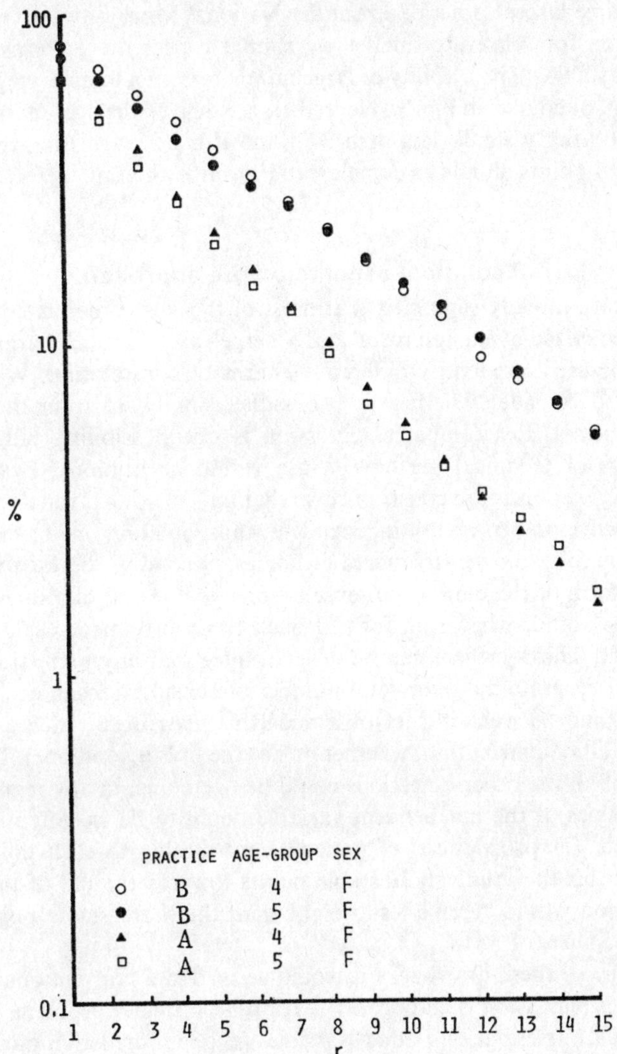

Figure 10. Observed proportion of patients consulting at least r times.

sex groups (though not in every practice), and that with one or two exceptions already mentioned most sets of points could reasonably adequately be represented, at least up to $r = 8$, by a straight line. One of the contributory factors to this must be that we have chosen the three largest practices from the National Morbidity Survey, and so even for relatively small r we should expect the patterns to be fairly stable. (The stability of large numbers is seen to an even greater extent, of course, in Fig. 3.) Nevertheless, some of the age–sex groups are still fairly small (less than 200) and it is not surprising that the plotted points should become erratic towards the tail.

Technical aspects of the approach

We have already suggested that most of the sets of points could be characterized by an 'intercept' and a 'slope', and that such parameters can be used to identify different patterns of consultation. We have now to consider whether it is possible, simply, to estimate these parameters. Least squares regression is one possibility, but for a variety of technical reasons its use would be dubious. First, the successive points are constrained so that $h(r) \geqslant h(r+1)$ for all $r \geqslant 1$; successive points are not independent, thus violating one of the conditions for valid least squares estimates. Secondly, the logarithmic transform of the data in no sense ensures that the fit of a line to the points would, when transformed back to an arithmetic scale, be a best fit. Thirdly, there can be no guarantee that any regression line would generate the same total number of consultations in each age–sex group as were in fact observed (this *must* occur with a fitted probability distribution, whether or not the fit is a good one). Lastly, even if all the other objections could be overcome, in any regression the values of the independent variable ought to be weighted by the number (or proportion) of patients contributing to each point. In doing this the relatively unstable points towards the tail of the distribution would receive less weight than the more stable points at lower values of r.

With all these drawbacks it would seem that a conventional least squares regression is inappropriate for this particular problem. There are, of course, various other possible methods for deriving a slope and an intercept. For example, Sadovski (6) has given a Fortran algorithm for computing α and β when it is desired to minimize the mean absolute deviation

$$\frac{1}{n} \sum_{i=1}^{n} \left| y_i - \alpha - \beta x_i \right|.$$

However, whatever analytical approach it is desired to use, we must reiterate that the search is for a simple method of comparison of patterns of usage in different groups of people both within and between practices. The method of least squares may be a slightly more widely understood technique (in terms of how to do it) than fitting a negative binomial distribution, but it is still very doubtful if many GPs would contemplate using it at all, even were it theoretically correct to do so. The same point has to be made, with greater emphasis, against the use of algorithms minimizing the mean absolute deviation or some similar expression. Indeed, the simplicity of our approach, which initially consists of plotting points on logarithmic graph paper, would be complicated by any attempt to reintroduce analytical methods at this stage. The final section therefore gives a more detailed exposition of our proposals.

Conclusion

We have shown that, for a variety of age and sex groups, a plot on logarithmic graph paper of the numbers of persons consulting at least once, at least twice, and so on within a given period of time, results in approximately a straight line, characterized by an intercept and slope. If the registered list size for a given subgroup is known, the points are easily expressed as a proportion of the list size, and the intercept corresponds to the proportion of registered patients consulting. The slope corresponds in some sense to a 'reconsultation rate', which can alternatively be expressed as the proportion of those patients consulting r times who return for a further consultation. It can therefore be regarded as a measure of 'chronicity'; for example a 'flat' slope indicates a relatively high reconsultation rate and identifies a group of high users of the GP services.

It is obvious that, for time-intervals larger than one year, the form of the distribution will change; the same holds for very short intervals. Certainly, the slopes and intercepts of curves based on different interval lengths will vary, and there may also be a departure from the approximate straight-line relationship. The method we propose is not, therefore, intended as a totally general one: it is offered as a simple and pragmatic procedure suitable for annual review procedures.

Figs. 5–10 demonstrate different types of practice usage for several subgroups of the practices considered. Fig. 6 is an example of two age-groups where there is a contrast between the sexes in that the pattern for females has a 'flatter' slope than that for males; the explanation for this contrast is the obstetric, gynaecological, and psychiatric conditions occurring in women in these age-groups, which involve frequent repeat consultations. Thus there is a recognizable biological basis for this contrast, as there is in Fig. 5 where a contrast between ages 0–4 and 5–14 is shown, but not between the sexes.

Perhaps what is more interesting from a management viewpoint are the contrasts shown in Figs. 8–10. These last three diagrams all pose the question of why patients in practice B should, apparently at least, receive 'more' service from their GP than those in practices A and C. Clearly additional information, such as the doctor–patient ratios, would be needed even to begin to answer such a question; our method at least demonstrates that there *are* differences and that it could be of practical importance to discover the reasons for them.

It might be objected that the above contrasts between sexes, between ages and between practices are reflected in the simple consultation rate. However, as has been demonstrated in Fig. 4, equal rates can conceal quite different patterns of consultation, and it may be important in managerial terms to distinguish between the patterns as well as the over-all amount of consultation. Another point, discussed in the introduction, was that the consultation rate requires a consistent and uniquely defined denominator, which is difficult to obtain in situations of population mobility. To the extent that all the foregoing diagrams have been presented in terms of 'the proportion of patients consulting at least r times', and are thus also dependent upon a defined population size, this particular criticism of the consultation rate is unfounded. However, it is possible to obviate the 'defined denominator' problem by our method, whereas with the consultation rate it is not.

Instead of calculating the proportion of patients consulting at least r times, we begin with the crude *numbers* consulting at least r times. Since the sizes of age, sex, and practice groups differ widely, merely plotting numbers would identify 'intercepts' mostly reflecting the absolute sizes of the particular groups concerned. If, instead, the numbers were transformed so that the measure for all persons consulting at least once were (say) 1,000, subsequent points for the same group would be derived by multiplication of each of the numbers by a simple proportion. This would enable a comparison to be made between the slopes of the consulting patterns for any groups desired, and could be used even in a non-NHS context where patients are not registered with GPs. To sum up, where population sizes *are* known, the consultation rate may be misleading; and where they are *not* known, so that consultation rates cannot be calculated, our method can still be used. The method proposed above involves counting the number of patients who consult their GP at least once, at least twice and so on, within a given period of time. As far as we know, such a recording process is not routinely carried out by GPs, but we suggest that it could easily be implemented in the operational setting of general practice with little clerical effort. Clearly, numerous refinements could be made depending upon the particular interest of the doctors concerned; for example, separate records could be kept of consultations made by males and females, by patients in different age-groups, or in combinations of these or other medico-social variables of interest. Care is needed to ensure that the sizes of the subgroups chosen are not so small as to give rise to wild fluctuations in the plotted points; groups with less than about 200 persons consulting may be unsatisfactory in this respect.

We thank Dr D. L. Crombie for making available data from the National Morbidity Survey.

References

1. ASHFORD, J. R. (1972). 'Patient contacts in general practice in the National Health Service', *The Statistician,* **21,** 265–89.
2. —— and HUNT, R. G. (1974). 'The distribution of doctor–patient contacts in the National Health Service', *Jl R. Statist. Soc.* **A 137,** 347–83.
3. FARMER, R. D. T., KNOX, E. G., CROSS, K. W., and CROMBIE, D. L. (1974). 'Executive Council lists and general practitioner files', *Br. J. prev. soc. Med.* **28,** 49–53.
4. FROGGATT, P., DUDGEON, M. G., and MERRETT, J. D. (1969). 'Consultation in general practice. Analysis of individual frequencies', ibid. **23,** 1–11.
5. OPCS (1974). *Morbidity Statistics from General Practice. Second National Study, 1970–71.* Studies on Medical and Population Subjects, no. 26 (London: HMSO).
6. SADOVSKI, A. N. (1974). 'L1-norm fit of a straight line. Algorithm AS 74', *Applied Statistics,* **23,** 244–8.
7. SPENCER, P. (1971). *General Practice and Models of the Referral Process.* Institute for Operational Research Health Reports no. 6 (Tavistock Institute of Human Relations).

Mathematical appendix

In this appendix we examine the nature of the data transformation described in the text and demonstrate that the resulting distribution is log–linear, or at least approximately so.

If x is the number of consultations made by an individual in one year, then

$$f(x) = \binom{x+w-1}{x} p^w q^x \quad x = 0, 1, 2 \dots$$

and p and w are the parameters of the negative binomial distribution. (1)

$$\text{Define} \quad g(r) = \sum_{x=r}^{\infty} \binom{x+w-1}{x} p^w q^x \quad r = 1, 2, 3 \dots$$

$$\text{then} \quad g(1) = 1-p^w$$

$$g(2) = 1-p^w-\binom{w}{1} qp^w \tag{2}$$

etc.

It should be noted that 'patients' failing to make any contact at all, ie persons registered with a practice but not consulting within it, are excluded from further consideration.

$$\text{Let} \quad h(r) = \frac{g(r)}{\sum\limits_{r=1}^{\infty} g(r)} \tag{3}$$

then $h(r)$ is a density, since $\sum\limits_{r=1}^{\infty} h(r) = 1$.

The new distribution can be described in one of two ways: as the distribution of the number of patients making at least r contacts during the year; or as the distribution of the 'rank' r of each consultation made (for example, if a person comes to see a GP for the 10th time, the consultation is one of 'rank' 10. There are, unfortunately, statistical connotations in the use of this word 'rank', connotations which we expressly wish to avoid. 'Rank' is used in a sense different from its common usage in order statistics). Rewriting (3) in full.

$$h(r) = \frac{\sum\limits_{x=r}^{\infty} \binom{x+w-1}{x} p^w q^x}{\sum\limits_{r=1}^{\infty} \sum\limits_{x=r}^{\infty} \binom{x+w-1}{x} p^w q^x}$$

$$= \frac{\dfrac{1}{\Gamma(w)} \sum\limits_{x=r}^{\infty} \dfrac{q^x}{x!} \Gamma(x+w)}{\dfrac{1}{\Gamma(w)} \sum\limits_{r=1}^{\infty} \sum\limits_{x=r}^{\infty} \dfrac{q^w}{x!} \Gamma(x+w)}$$

$$= \frac{\sum\limits_{x=r}^{\infty} \dfrac{q^x}{x!} \Gamma(x+w)}{\sum\limits_{r=1}^{\infty} \sum\limits_{x=r}^{\infty} \dfrac{q^x}{x!} \Gamma(x+w)} \tag{4}$$

The denominator of (4) is a constant, and hence

$$h(r) = K. \sum\limits_{x=r}^{\infty} \dfrac{q^x}{x!} \Gamma(x+w)$$

whose successive terms may be written as follows:

$$h(1) = K\left[q.w! + \frac{q^2}{2!}(w+1)! + \frac{q^3}{3!}(w+2)! + \ldots \right] \tag{5[i]}$$

$$h(2) = K\left[\frac{q^2}{2!}(w+1)! + \frac{q^3}{3!}(w+2)! + \ldots \right] \tag{[ii]}$$

$$h(3) = K\left[\frac{q^3}{3!}(w+2)! + \ldots \right]. \tag{[iii]}$$

The value of w is clearly of critical importance in determining the numerical properties of these terms. Consider first the special case of $w = 1$.

$$\text{Then} \quad h(1) = K. \sum_{r=1}^{\infty} q^r = K.\frac{q}{p}$$

$$h(2) = K.\frac{q^2}{p}$$

$$h(3) = K.\frac{q^3}{p}$$

etc.

If the constant K is evaluated, $h(r)$ becomes the geometric distribution pq^{r-1}, with successive terms in geometric progression. On logarithmic graph paper, the terms of $h(r)$ form a straight line whose slope is inversely proportional to q, and whose intercept (at $r = 1$) can be used to represent either the proportion of a registered list size who consult at all, or (particularly in a non-NHS context), simply the number of persons visiting a doctor at least once during a year. The use of the data in these forms is discussed in more detail in the main text.

For $w \neq 1$, the approximation to a geometric progression can be investigated in two ways. Firstly, we have a g.p. (and hence log-linearity) if the ratio of the rth to the $(r+1)$th term is constant for all $r \geqslant 1$, ie if

$$\frac{h(r)}{h(r+1)} = C, \text{ say} \tag{6}$$

It is easier, however, to consider the second method of showing the existence of a g.p., namely, that the logarithms of the difference of adjacent terms shall be in arithmetic progression, ie, that $\log[h(2)-h(1)]$, $\log\,[h(3)-h(2)]$, $\log\,[h(4)-h(3)]$, etc., are in arithmetic progression. From equations 5[i]–[iii], we have

$$h(2)-h(1) = K.q\,w!$$

$$h(3)-h(2) = K.\frac{q^2}{2!}(w+1)!$$

$$h(4)-h(3) = K.\frac{q^3}{3!}(w+2)!$$

so that

$$\log [h(2)-h(1)] = \log q+\log (w!)+\log K \tag{7[i]}$$

$$\log [h(3)-h(2)] = 2 \log q-\log 2+\log (w+1)+\log (w!)+\log K \tag{ii}$$

$$\log [h(4)-h(3)] = 3 \log q-\log 3-\log 2+\log (w+2)+\\ \log (w+1)+\log (w!)+\log K. \tag{iii}$$

The first terms of each of these expressions are in arithmetic progression and the last two terms are identical. The departure from an a.p. (ie log-linearity) depends on the middle terms, which are represented by the expression

$$\sum_{r=2}^{n} \log (w+r-1)- \sum_{r=2}^{n} \log r \tag{8}$$

in the *n*th term of equation 7 (for $n > 1$). The closer w is to 1, then the nearer is the above expression to zero, the closer successive terms of equation (7) are to an arithmetic progression and the closer $h(r)$ comes to being a geometric progression. When $w < 1$, it can also be seen from (8) that

$$\sum_{r=2}^{n} \log (w+r-1) < \sum_{r=2}^{n} \log r \text{ for all } n \geqslant 2,$$

ie the middle terms become increasingly negative, and the line joining the points $\log [h(r)]$ is thus convex from below. Conversely, when $w > 1$ the middle terms become increasingly positive and the line is concave from below. Examples of this can be seen in Fig. A1, in which points are plotted for combinations of q and w which roughly represent the extreme values of these parameters estimated in the main paper.

Finally, each additional term of (8) incorporates an increment (or decrement) of $\log (w+n-1)-\log n$, representing the additional departure of the corresponding term of (7) from an arithmetic progression. For a given value of w in the range $0 < w < 2$ (which easily encompasses the range of estimated ws) and for $w \neq 1$, $\log (w+n-1)-\log n$ is greater when n is small than when n is large.

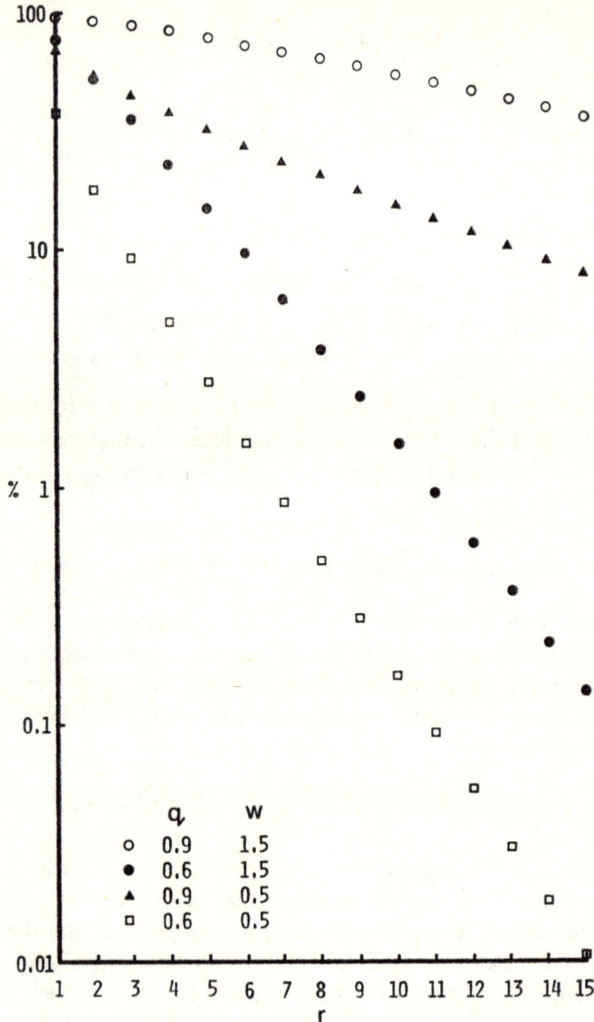

Figure A1. Theoretical proportion of patients consulting at least *r* times.

Hence the theoretical approximation to linearity is better towards the tail of the distribution (that is, when the negative binomial is the appropriate functional form of $f(x)$), though in practice it is in the tail that the number of patients concerned is usually small and their distribution is likely to be erratic.

The 'improving linearity' of the theoretical expression is well demonstrated in Fig. A1, where only the first two or three terms show any substantial departure from linearity. It is clear, though, that in the approximately linear region, the 'slope' of the line is not proportional (inversely or otherwise) to q alone (as it is when $w = 1$), but depends also on w. It is difficult to formulate any analytical rules for assessing whether the theoretical approximation of $h(r)$ to a geometric progression is in some sense adequate. We have shown that, for a particular functional form, the approximation will be 'quite close'; but the utility of the method must be assessed on heuristic grounds by examining the original data, whether or not the negative binomial is appropriate.

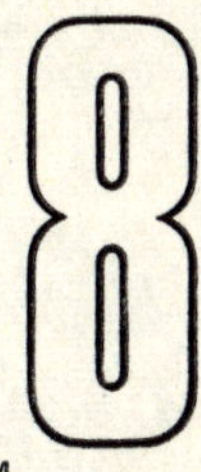

E. G. Knox
MD, FRCP, FFCM,
Health Services Research Centre
Department of Social Medicine
University of Birmingham

Security standards for computer medical records

Security standards for computer medical records

Introduction

There is some public concern over the confidentiality and security of medical (and other personal) records. Computer methods provoke special comment, although justifiable worries are probably more appropriate to handwritten than to magnetic records. It is certainly less easy to be careless with computer records than with traditional ones and casual access is relatively difficult for unauthorized and unskilled people. Nevertheless we must take public worries seriously and demonstrate this fact by identifying and eliminating the security risks, if for no other reason than to protect record automation developments (and the services and benefits which depend upon them) from the obstructions which this kind of anxiety can engender.

This is not simply a question of extending current record-handling practices (which would be regarded as grossly sub-standard in any computer-usage context) into a new technical field; the problem is different in kind. Unauthorized access to computer files is necessarily deliberate rather than casual, depends upon skill rather than carelessness, may require some investment, and is quite likely to be motivated maliciously, or for purposes at variance with the best interests of the patient or the intention of the doctor who recorded the information. Furthermore, theft might be attempted on a considerable scale. Any security system whatsoever must protect records of previously identified persons against individual search and scrutiny (for example, for personal, blackmail, legal, purposes), but there is a special need with computer records to defeat the intentions of persons who wish to use whole files for commercial or even predatory purposes or for large-scale linkage operations connected with purposes outside the legitimate field of medical practice and authorized research (for example, linking alcoholic histories or diagnoses of epilepsy with driving licence applications; or sickness records with insurance proposals, claims for sickness benefit, or job suitability assessments). In addition, an ideal system should protect its guardian from subpoena or other irresistible instructions to betray confidentiality.

The security problems of the two kinds of records differ also in the types of protective mechanism which are appropriate and effective. Traditional security problems are met in large part by the use of words. That is, the importance of the duty of secrecy is passed by word of mouth between those concerned in handling records, it is reinforced by explicit professional standards (for example, of Hippocrates, British Computer Society, etc.), is backed by verbally stated or written rules restraining the release or movement of records, and is enforced where necessary through an explicit or implicit hierarchy or accountability from clerks and secretaries through supervisors to nurses, doctors, administrators, and other staff in charge. Accountability terminates ultimately in sanctions related to continued employment, continued registration, or in the courts. It is difficult in a highly manned record-handling system to gain access to records without the co-operation of an aware and wary staff; the whole system is reinforced by talking about it. Quite simple additional procedures can provide considerable enhancements of protection against illicit accession; for example, the commendable practice of keeping records in a non-alphabetical order, thus requiring the additional step of looking up sequence numbers in an index (which can be locked away), can make things very difficult for the thief who breaks and enters, or who for other reason has only a short time at his disposal.

Protection mechanisms of these kinds are also necessary in relation to computer systems, and particularly with respect to printed outputs, coded inputs, and magnetic tape libraries.

We must recognize, however, that such processes may not be sufficient and that a determined and skilful attack on any standard medical records system would have a reasonable chance of succeeding: as a notorious political example has shown. Even an isolated breakage can amount to a very serious failure from the point of view of the system. Because medical records on magnetic media are the ones which seem to cause the greatest public anxieties, and because they are the ones which for technical reasons are most susceptible to 'mass' theft, they deserve the protection of relatively elaborate encipherment practices and authorization traps.

Finally, if for no other purpose than the public reassurance which might be provided, it is necessary to define and set acceptable and practicable operational standards for our security practices. Through reference to such standards it would then be possible to make explicit the level of security being offered in a particular situation, whether the reference standard is accepted entire, or whether it is modified by relaxations or enhancements thought necessary in the particular context.

This is the subject of this paper; it contributes an analysis of the various security problems which arise in relation to computer medical records, suggests methods of overcoming them, investigates their implementation, and proposes a set of operational standards to cover the most important security practices.

THE NATURE OF THE PROBLEM

Computer records are held on magnetic media such as tapes, discs, or cards. This in itself supplies a degree of security in that most magnetic media require special environmental conditions for their storage, usually in a computer unit. This is often, although not necessarily, a reasonably secure place. In addition, a computer is necessary for their interpretation. However, it would be difficult to guarantee that such media could never be stolen or copied illicitly, or sequestered through some legal or other authoritative mechanism (for example through ownership of the computer or the magnetic media themselves). Once so obtained, computer records may be printed out literally on a wide variety of computers using general programs on whose usage there are no effective constraints.

Degrees of protection can be provided by the removal of personal identities when the purpose does not require them; they are not always necessary for research or service review purposes or for statistical file analysis. Data other than identities can often be 'coded' in the sense that meanings are represented by single characters or short groups of characters rather than plain text. However, records used for scheduling medical care are generally useless without identities, and codes can often be interpreted fairly accurately by an experienced person; in many cases they will be standard codes such as numerical diagnostic codes, which are readily available. In addition, certain kinds of research require identities as well as medical data, for example to ensure against duplication of records, or to link records made on different dates into a common sequence, or to link children into sibships, or for similar purposes. A suitable security practice must cover all these circumstances. Therefore, whenever records contain both medical data and specific identities, or data from which identification could be made indirectly, the question reduces itself to one of 'encipherment'. By 'encipherment' we imply a character-for-character substitution, as opposed to the character-for-meaning substitution implied by the term 'coding'.

Encipherment, and its inverse decipherment, are normally carried out by a computer program using 'keys' to which access must be restricted. Encipherment/decipherment practices are dependent for their security upon the authorization practices which go with them, and the analysis which follows in this paper is concerned with these two themes.

ENCIPHERMENT AND DECIPHERMENT

A satisfactory encipherment method reorders and/or substitutes the characters of the original message so that no meaning is immediately evident. A satisfactory system should be resistant to cracking through the analysis of character frequencies or through clues arising from the tendency of medical records to have a stereotyped structure. For example the initial digits of six-digit serial-numbers in the early parts of records change infrequently, certain areas of records tend to be numeric and others alphabetical, and variable-length records fitted into fixed-length record-areas result in a regular concentration of blank spaces in certain parts of the record-area. Ciphers can also be cracked by comparing successive versions and analysing the effects of inserting new records to a file, or new elements to a record, and a satisfactory system should resist this kind of approach. An ideal system should not only neutralize the theft of a file or of several files but also the theft of other parts of the system. It should be impossible, for example, to decipher a record separated from its file, even though the program and authorization are available; it should be impossible to follow the detailed working of a stolen program without the simultaneous theft of the file and the authorization key; it should be impossible to short-circuit the authorization mechanism of a stolen program and proceed successfully to the decipherment process. Every part of the system should be so interdependent that nothing short of total sequestration would enable data to be accessed. Finally, the process should be reasonably economic.

It is evident that cipher systems using constant character-for-character substitutions do not meet any of these requirements. The use of a look-up matrix in both directions for every character may prove prohibitive in programming time and the result is very susceptible to character frequency analysis. Once the key-matrix has been deduced, all authorization constraints can be bypassed. Direct logical operations upon the binary patterns of computer-stored characters are better. For example, the use of binary complementation techniques, substituting 0 for 1 and 1 for 0, are much more economical in computer time. However, binary complementation is as susceptible to cracking through character frequency analysis as the results of using a look-up matrix and would not even have the advantage that the matrix could be changed.

A more satisfactory method is the modulo-2 addition method. Modulo-2 addition is carried out with binary bit patterns, either character by character, or byte by byte, or word by word. The binary message is set against a binary key and the cipher is constructed on the basis that where the key and message are the same (0,0 or 1,1) then the cipher is set 0, while where the key and message differ (0,1 or 1,0) the cipher is set as 1. In effect, it consists in 'casting out' pairs of '1s' in each column. This technique shares with binary complementation the advantage that a second application regenerates the message thus:

Message	0 0 0 1 1 1 0 1
Key	1 0 1 0 1 0 1 0
	———————
Cipher	1 0 1 1 0 1 1 1
Key	1 0 1 0 1 0 1 0
	———————
Message	0 0 0 1 1 1 0 1

In both the binary complementation method and in the modulo-2 method the actual written character transformation depends upon the character-code-set of the computer. Binary complementation is in fact exactly equivalent to the modulo-2 method using a key consisting entirely of '1s'. The modulo-2 method will thus permit the key to be changed from time to time, but if used constantly throughout, a record or file should be soluble through character frequency analysis within a matter of minutes.

The only systems which are reasonably secure from character frequency analysis are those which use non-constant substitutions. The true value of the modulo-2 method is that it lends itself to this kind of operation and its power appears when we add the step of using the cipher produced by one operation, as the key to the next. Thus, in a series of n words, word $n-1$ may be used to encode word n, and word $n-2$ may be used to encode word $n-1$, and so on until word 1 encodes word 2. Finally, the whole sequence can be locked using an external key to encode word 1. In this way every word is transformed and every key is hidden. Decipherment is accomplished in the reverse order.

This system is theoretically resistant to character frequency analysis and in continuous text this is effectively true (Feistel, 1973). However, a code-cracker who suspected the general method might be able to make use of the stereotyped structures of medical records, as discussed earlier. A simple and reasonably satisfactory solution is to start the process somewhere in the middle of the record rather than at one end and to conduct the encipherment sequence by skipping several records, rather than on the basis of adjacency. For example, if a record consisting of 80 characters were entered at character 10, this enciphered by using record 17, and this one using record 24 and so on in steps of 7 (re-entering to the beginning of the record when character 80 had been passed), the would-be code-cracker would certainly have a more difficult job. If the chosen stepping frequency is a prime number which does not divide exactly into the record length then the full set of words or characters can be covered in the same number of operations as those used in a simple sequential pattern.

It is possible in addition to use entry points and/or stepping numbers which vary from record to record and from generation to generation of the file and are some reproducible function of the sequence number of the record within the file and of a file-sequence number, and perhaps of a numerical constant released by the user-authorization process. Thus, if a file is read, updated by the insertion or deletion of a record, or of material within records, then the two files should show no recognizable resemblances between their earlier and later enciphered versions. For example, we might base the entry point upon the record sequence number and file sequence number, while the stepping frequency and the locking key could be based upon an interaction between authorization keys and some additional data held in the program itself and in the initial block of the file. Elaborations of this degree are probably desirable in order to confuse the code-cracker who obtained a sequential pair of files. These elaborations should be designed to defeat the ability of the code-cracker to exploit a weakness of the modulo-2 system, namely that when the binary operation is carried out on the message and the cipher, it generates the key.

In practical trials, however, this system reveals an unexpected defect. This is illustrated in Fig. 1 where successive encipherments of the same message, using different entry points, but the same stepping pattern, are laid out side by side. The successive encipherments turn out to be surprisingly similar. In retrospect this is because each word is enciphered by the same key, except for the point of closure by the external locking key. It would therefore be quite easy for a code-cracker to discover which items on one generation of a file corresponded with which items on the second. Furthermore, he could very quickly deduce the stepping frequency from the differences, and he could very simply regenerate the closure key. He could probably also infer the entry point rule. In any circumstances where two successive files could be stolen, as in many tape-file systems, this particular method could not be relied upon.

An alternative approach is to apply the encipherment/decipherment principles referred to earlier, in an inverse manner. That is, encipherment is accomplished by entry to the record with the 'closure' key, the result of which is used to encipher another word, the result of that another word, and so on. Decipherment would then be practised in reverse order. This method has the disadvantage that the keys are not obscured and remain within the enciphered record. On the other hand it has the great advantage that confusion is propagated through the message with the result that successive versions really do bear no resemblance to each other. This is illustrated in Fig. 2. With this method a change in the 'closure' key also changes the outcome entirely, whereas with the earlier method, it changes only one word at the point of exit, and it reveals both its location and its identity. No one could ever guarantee that a forward-encipherment system of the kind illustrated in Fig. 2 could *never* be cracked, but it would certainly be exceedingly difficult by any intuitive methods, would probably require expensive and difficult computer analysis procedures, and all in all offers a very high level of security for a very limited additional cost in computer time. The additional computation would in most cases constitute a very small fraction of the waiting time between record reading operations in most magnetic tape or magnetic disc systems. Additional security, sufficient to obstruct even an expert crypto-analyst, can be obtained by repeated encipherment using different orders and different keys.

```
TEST MFSSAGE FOR FNCODF/DFCODE PROGRAM. ALTERNATE ENCODING/DECODING.
T.F#G89.MA!>T]21A'‡C(]\@ 1>&![FZ2>31!S.T9? E8‡*09G N[ YI‡,£>[!= 1>&2E
TEST MFSSAGE FOR FNCODF/DFCODE PROGRAM. ALTERNATE ENCODING/DECODING.
T.F#G89.MA!>T]21A'‡C(¤!= 1>&![FZ2>31!S.T9? E8‡*0!B9N[ YI‡,£>[!= 1>&2E
TEST MFSSAGE FOR FNCODF/DFCODE PROGRAM. ALTERNATE ENCODING/DECODING.
T.F#G8!@*A!>T]21A'‡C(¤!= 1>&![FZ2>31!S.T9? E8‡*09G N[ YI‡,£>[!= 1>&2E
TEST MFSSAGE FOR ENCODF/DFCODE PROGRAM. ALTERNATE ENCODING/DECODING.
T.F#G89.MA!>T]21A'‡C(¤!= 1>&![FZ2¤[V!S.T9? E8‡*09G N[ YI‡,£>[!= 1>&2E
TEST MFSSAGE FOR ENCODF/DFCODE PROGRAM. ALTERNATE ENCODING/DECODING.
T.F#G89.MA!>T]21A'‡C(¤!= 1>&![FZ2>31!S.T9? E8‡*09G N[ YI‡,£>!0) 1>&2E
TEST MFSSAGE FOR FNCODE/DFCODE PROGRAM. ALTERNATE ENCODING/DECODING.
T.F#G89.MA!>T]21A'>0)¤!= 1>&![FZ2>31!S.T9? E8‡*09G N[ YI‡,£>[!= 1>&2E
TEST MFSSAGE FOR FNCODF/DFCODE PROGRAM. ALTERNATE ENCODING/DECODING.
T.F#G89.MA!>T]21A'‡C(¤!= 1>&![FZ2>31!S.T9? E8>]£9G N[ YI‡,£>[!= 1>&2E
TEST MFSSAGE FOR FNCODF/DFCODE PROGRAM. ALTERNATE ENCODING/DECODING.
T.F@B&9.MA!>T]21A'‡C(¤!= 1>&![FZ2>31!S.T9? E8‡*09G N[ YI‡,£>[!= 1>&2E
TEST MFSSAGE FOR ENCODF/DFCODE PROGRAM. ALTERNATE ENCODING/DECODING.
T.F#G89.MA!>T]21A'‡C(¤!= 1>&![C¤V>31!S.T9? E8‡*09G N[ YI‡,£>[!= 1>&2E
TEST MFSSAGE FOR FNCODF/DFCODE PROGRAM. ALTERNATE ENCODING/DECODING.
T.F#G89.MA!>T]21A'‡C(¤!= 1>&![FZ2>31!S.T9? E8‡*09G N[ YI‡9*0[!= 1>&2E
TEST MFSSAGE FOR ENCODE/DFCODE PROGRAM. ALTERNATE ENCODING/DECODING.
T.F#G89.MA!>T]2XA9‡C(¤!= 1>&![FZ;>31!S.T9? E8‡*09G N[ YI‡,£>[!= 1>&2E
TEST MFSSAGE FOR ENCODF/DFCODE PFOGRAM. ALTERNATE ENCODING/DECODING.
T.F#G89.MA!>T]21A'‡C(¤!= 1>&![FZ2>31!S.T9?@\V‡*09G N[ YI‡,£>[!= 1>&2E
TEST MFSSAGE FOR ENCODF/DFCODE PROGRAM. ALTERNATE ENCODING/DECODING.
@\*#G89.MA!>T]21A'‡C(¤!= 1>&![FZ2>31!S.T9? E8‡*09G N[ YI‡,£>[!= 1>&2E
TEST MESSAGE FOR ENCODF/DFCODE PROGRAM. ALTERNATE ENCODING/DECODING.
T.F#G89.MA!>T]21A'‡C(¤!= 1>¤-9FZ2>31!S.T9? E8‡*09G N[ YI‡,£>[!= 1>&2F
TEST MFSSAGE FOR FNCODF/DFCODE PROGRAM. ALTERNATE ENCODING/DECODING.
T.F#G89.MA!>T]21A'‡C(¤!= 1>&![FZ2>31!S.T9? E8‡*09G N[ ]6Z,£>[!= 1>&2E
TEST MFSSAGE FOR FNCODF/DFCODE PROGRAM. ALTERNATE ENCODING/DECODING.
T.F#G89.MA!>C9)1A'‡C(¤!= 1>&![FZ2>31!S.T9? E8‡*09G N[ YI‡,£>[!= 1>&2E
TEST MFSSAGE FOR ENCODF/DFCODE PROGRAM. ALTERNATE ENCODING/DECODING.
T.F#G89.MA!>T]21A'‡C(¤!= ·1>&![FZ2>31!S.C], E8‡*09G N[ YI‡,£>[!= 1>&2E
TEST MFSSAGE FOR FNCODF/DFCODE PROGRAM. ALTERNATE ENCODING/DECODING.
T.F#G89.MA!>T]21A'‡C(¤!= 1>&![FZ2>31!S.T9? E8‡*09G N[ YI‡,£>[!= 1>94A
TEST MFSSAGE FOR ENCODF/DFCODE PROGRAM. ALTERNATE ENCODING/DECODING.
T.F#G89.MA!>T]21A'‡C(¤!=]\-&![FZ2>31!S.T9? E8‡*09G N[ YI‡,£>[!= 1>&2E
TEST MFSSAGE FOR FNCODF/DFCODE PROGRAM. ALTERNATE ENCODING/DECODING.
T.F#G89.MA!>T]21A'‡C(¤!= 1>&![FZ2>31!S.T9? E8‡*09G >0)YI‡,£>[!= 1>&2E
TEST MFSSAGE FOR FNCODF/DFCODE PROGRAM. ALTERNATE ENCODING/DECODING.
T.F#G89.M-[9T]21A'‡C(¤!= 1>&![FZ2>31!S.T9? E8‡*09G N[ YI‡,£>[!= 1>&2E
TEST MFSSAGE FOR FNCODF/DFCODE PROGRAM. ALTERNATE ENCODING/DECODING.
T.F#G89.MA!>T]21A'‡C(¤!= 1>&![FZ2>31-,3T9? E8‡*09G N[ YI‡,£>[!= 1>&2E
TEST MFSSAGE FOR FNCODF/DFCODE PROGRAM. ALTERNATE ENCODING/DECODING.
T.F#G89.MA!>T]21A'‡C(¤!= 1>&![FZ2>31!S.T9? E8‡*09G N[ YI‡,£>[!=]6Z&2F
```

Figure 1. Results of 'reverse' encoding procedure.

The algorithms responsible for the encipherments in the two figures are provided in Appendix 1. The subroutines are written in Fortran which in this case operates upon records assembled in the form of an array of 'INTEGERS' with three characters per word. This is an arrangement used on a Univac 418 and represents the form of a record immediately after reading into core from magnetic tape or disc, and immediately before writing to another. With very small changes it is equally applicable to storage in arrays of 'REALS' a more usual arrangement in other machines. The results in Fig. 1 were obtained by using the subroutines in an inverse order from that implied by their names.

```
TEST MESSAGE FOR ENCODE/DECODE PROGRAM. ALTERNATE ENCODING/DECODING.
^O+£11'.UYM'A2]P3F8(#]\QP-MV.+F(KA1!TM-Δ)TAIN33]!MT7.?N)G(:25FH6)<[£ +
TEST MESSAGE FOR ENCODE/DECODE PROGRAM. ALTERNATE ENCODING/DECODING.
N=C[T>nQ\Z?NWUY4/!LOK3WL4±=BQP<2!WTFHBVN6≠W'.Q/Y:B9:*.+N8ZU,<Δ[+RS[,P
TEST MESSAGE FOR ENCODE/DECODE PROGRAM. ALTERNATE ENCODING/DECODING.
K=X-T.:Q*(?1/UD7/[]2S8W77±(.LX?2[/TSZ?NK6I/'>L/DO?II*>=NMH(£?Δ!=RFN/X
TEST MESSAGE FOR ENCODE/DECODE PROGRAM. ALTERNATE ENCODING/DECODING.
'JU6[#^#+XP6¤:GQ8>7ZV  4Q[ W#UFZ-¤[VUPK'#:¤D&48L£P:DE&ZDC+5ΔEC'Z?N!\U
TEST MESSAGE FOR ENCODE/DECODE PROGRAM. ALTERNATE ENCODING/DECODING.
V(JSI≠W7nR¤GO=S)<%IOQZ?N)G?Δ7J:O:OID*¤TVK-01I:<S/¤-Q8IP-23=Z:0)P3YSFJ
TEST MESSAGE FOR ENCODE/DECODE PROGRAM. ALTERNATE ENCODING/DECODING.
±=:DTLHQRJ?±*U!#/Y>0)<W>#±2\Q,32Y*T]0BQ#6N*'7&/!Z?N6+75N?JUP3ΔD5R%D,,
TEST MESSAGE FOR ENCODE/DECODE PROGRAM. ALTERNATE ENCODING/DECODING.
)N[GOM7?NOL(R-£.]XF± ?9¤.?1P?[A±XRO JL=)ZORH8>]£(LO1A82=.O1D8GC2FR≠][
TEST MESSAGE FOR ENCODE/DECODE PROGRAM. ALTERNATE ENCODING/DECODING.
4>HQB&327?±KCAT-:.!LAOGQ-BR+2H(L'Z?N<±64P)C\#':78±)>-#B\XW.0(9-B617DH
TEST MESSAGE FOR ENCODE/DECODE PROGRAM. ALTERNATE ENCODING/DECODING.
QM\%7F*IP/O&H8IK511¤-J?]K9XUI\C¤VH7>WO#Q&QH.S65IROGA=S,AR<8BZ?N,+.%I\
TEST MESSAGE FOR ENCODE/DECODE PROGRAM. ALTERNATE ENCODING/DECODING.
E8M¤Q[ΛT79?F6*7U£.Z?NTΔDUI.RKTH'?.6QNQO6E#]6V!H£7A2]*U!Q>X9*0'W>QX1¤JH
TEST MESSAGE FOR ENCODE/DECODE PROGRAM. ALTERNATE ENCODING/DECODING.
RZW,D:A4<],41CAXR9(JTYF6X:,-4W'J91DT9,QBN#1[)Z?NF,#R )%6JQ+*!:Q%\GEBW
TEST MESSAGE FOR ENCODE/DECODE PROGRAM. ALTERNATE ENCODING/DECODING.
(>?Z?N±2HK±-QA:/:SBL&#G9/R8L2Z4L67?[N±'(PGQ\VE:%)±G5-V!\=[.J49K!6!ZD7
TEST MESSAGE FOR ENCODE/DECODE PROGRAM. ALTERNATE ENCODING/DECODING.
Q\*%QS*T3/O#H*±K£N1B'JΛ%KI CUT*7?NHQ.WO&QF4HVF6£±RO4&UF,> <*WZW1,X>%J*
TEST MESSAGE FOR ENCODE/DECODE PROGRAM. ALTERNATE ENCODING/DECODING.
-¤±KAEO-QC(:?B=%C?LM¤RH %.Y¤-9/M2?A¤(U<-QC?9/]C=:(CYO/X7%Z?N/\OX:?K+9
TEST MESSAGE FOR ENCODE/DECODE PROGRAM. ALTERNATE ENCODING/DECODING.
WZ*<D6V43%,#NC9Z?N=J'DF:C:P'4*Γ JAND'Q,&WN4N[K+?±S,4  K]6Z4+W[:V]\-/B*
TEST MESSAGE FOR ENCODE/DECODE PROGRAM. ALTERNATE ENCODING/DECODING.
4L+7813=U?N'C9)-6F!>#O-Q-\M+=+(>KZ8!<N-4,TZ?N'6]8NT>GABB(W75(A6B:[7[+
TEST MESSAGE FOR ENCODE/DECODE PROGRAM. ALTERNATE ENCODING/DECODING.
?7?NHV D'R-HP%W2?X=,\H.UE?>!]'A78=%VM[H3C],%QR¤X2GH,2ΔR1LSNW97*(1£8H7A
TEST MESSAGE FOR ENCODE/DECODE PROGRAM. ALTERNATE ENCODING/DECODING.
QNN90  B¤L CX-21]=[≠M29E1?!Z?N=±=X0MEQ3QZ:XHRN]2ML:,AR?=SB1±=G(?F894A
TEST MESSAGE FOR ENCODE/DECODE PROGRAM. ALTERNATE ENCODING/DECODING.
'Q668*^H'X'U¤7JQΓ 7V3 1W]\-WH6FVZ#83U'H'/Δ¤?\4[E£'ΔDI\Z?N+9:E.+C:P!66
TEST MESSAGE FOR ENCODE/DECODE PROGRAM. ALTERNATE ENCODING/DECODING.
4¤W7.%31<?(4Z?N-+±!MTOH6-A:+1W(M9Z.7<(Q4Q#Z7]'+N8(#>0)B9EW?*(\QB5L7CW
TEST MESSAGE FOR ENCODE/DECODE PROGRAM. ALTERNATE ENCODING/DECODING.
Z4:HRLDXR-[9%%!?'Y,F).!>?P?]X,7#Y%R][[QZ?N%/7¤'!G[A?Y71,?N%P7SD1T%HN,
TEST MESSAGE FOR ENCODE/DECODE PROGRAM. ALTERNATE ENCODING/DECODING.
(XNC: G4&K/CQ+2<?=B£M#<E<D!L]N4£=Q:M-,3('IQ6R,?2)/:53R6[S[C#45(68&Z?N
TEST MESSAGE FOR ENCODE/DECODE PROGRAM. ALTERNATE ENCODING/DECODING.
WV#<?UVOV%T*N.,ZDC=Q+DTΔZ?N'O#ΓQPN?+QT\WRWN8H+D:STW 1HQ8>4A4[73]67/:#
```

Figure 2. Results of 'forward' encoding procedure.

AUTHORIZATION METHODS

The actions for which authorization might be required include the
addition or deletion of records to and from a file, the addition or
deletion of contents to and from a record, the alteration of existing
material through a combination of deletion and addition, and simple
inspection of deciphered material.

Addition and deletion operations are normally subjected to quite
elaborate checks, not so much from the point of view of confidentiality as of careless operation. The details of these checks depend
upon the type of system in use, and particularly whether real-time

or batch-processing techniques are used. In real-time systems the files are protected from corruption by complex branching displays offering a limited choice of action, and all operations are logged by the system and can be displayed at will and attributed to their originators. The most serious weaknesses here occur when authorized users are careless with authorization keys or when they delegate their authority. For batch systems it is necessary to be sure that the file to be updated is the intended one, that the operation has not already been carried out by someone else, that the latest operation on this file has in fact been carried out as it is believed to have been, and that the alteration to be carried out belongs properly to this occasion and not to another one. File identification, file-generation, sequence-number, dates, and the identification and validity of new data are checked in all details.

All these operations are necessarily carried out under the close control of computer staffs and are therefore covered by the traditional 'human' systems referred to earlier. Illegal inspections of material *in situ* are therefore difficult, and the chief problems arise with respect to files which are intended to be (or can be) 'demounted' such as magnetic tapes.

These circumstances occur frequently, for example where periodic analysis and review of material is required, or where a file is updated regularly through a cycle of eight or ten magnetic tapes: to permit the operation of error recovery processes when data errors are discovered within a reasonably short time. Demountable files, if they are to be protected at all, must carry their own authorization keys.

Appendix 2 exemplifies an approach to this problem, again in the form of an algorithm written in Fortran and based upon the assumption that a magnetic data file would contain at its beginning a 'header-block' which would interact with the program and with input authorization keys (for example on cards). In this example an input key-card would contain three elements, (1) an address point within the header block from which the operation can begin, (2) a key for unlocking an area of the header block through the modulo-2 method, and (3) an authorization key to be compared with a set of options stored in this area. Unless the authorization key matches one of the stored keys the program will proceed no further. The authorization process cannot be short-circuited, because an interaction between stored elements and input elements is necessary in order to generate keys for unlocking individual records.

In addition to the normal user-key matching process, the header block contains an enciphered guardian-key. If this is matched successfully in an appropriate field of the authorization card, it permits alteration of the user-key matching set, of the entry point to the header block, of the cipher key for the header block, of the record decipherment closure-and-stepping-keys, and of the guardian key itself. The record closure key is not actually stored anywhere within the header block, within the program, or on the authorization card; it is constructed on each occasion through interactions between elements held in all three sites.

Obviously, this is a very tricky puzzle for anyone lacking any single element. Quite small modifications of the algorithm provided could successfully confuse a thief who had access to the principles upon which the general procedure operates, for example, this paper. In addition, the system could be used to defend its guardian against authoritarian instructions to betray confidentiality through the unrecorded alteration of the authorization keys. Alternatively, since resetting the authorization keys does not automatically delete the previous set (unless one set over-writes the other) it is possible to set up two separated alternative pathways within the same header block, one officially 'current' and one officially 'obsolete' or even un-declared. A number of 'accidental' interactions between two systems can be envisaged which would permit a valid exit from the authoriza-tion procedure, but with nonsense keys. A skilful programmer could readily incorporate a number of other cryptic key corruption mechanisms. Tertiary or quaternary levels of authorization and re-authorization could also be incorporated, perhaps without mention in the generally available specifications.

STANDARD SECURITY REQUIREMENTS

On the basis of the considerations presented and the implementations tested, it is possible to define a set of draft standards of security practice for computer records. They are presented below. They are intended neither as minima at one end of a scale, nor ideals at the other, but as a simple and economic reference standard. It should therefore be possible for a systems designer to say that he undertakes to meet these standards, or to meet standards no less stringent, or to meet standards with such and such an enhancement, or with such and such a relaxation.

1. All computer records containing personal identifications and

medical material should be enciphered in a form whose meaning is not self-evident.

2. The encipherment of medical records should depend upon character-for-character substitutions using a non-constant key, for example through a process using chained modulo-2 addition.

3. The encipherment mechanism should obscure the intrinsic stereotypy of medical records and should vary both from record to record within a file, and from copy to copy of the same file, and should depend for its entry point, its sequence and its closure, upon keys external to the record.

4. External record encipherment keys and sequence parameters should depend jointly upon the file itself, the encipherment/decipherment program and user-authorization keys, in such a way that the system is neither usable nor comprehensible without access to all of them simultaneously.

5. The encipherment system must depend for its operation upon an authorization mechanism such that bypassing the latter will prevent the decipherment system from working. Authorization keys must be issued by a file-guardian who must be provided with a means of cancelling and reissuing encipherment and authorization keys, including his own.

6. The user authorization reissue procedure should incorporate a cryptic key-corruption or file-corruption mechanism capable of blocking subsequent usage of the system in a manner so obscure and complex as to protect the guardian from accusations of engineering it deliberately.

Discussion

The main purpose of this section is to comment on the sixth draft standard under a separate heading. The standard invokes a circular argument in that a declaration of having met all six standards might itself expose a file-guardian or programmer to just such an accusation as that from which the standard seeks to protect. The question arises whether a suitable form of reference to the draft standard might be devised.

A systems designer might take one of three actions. He might declare that he had in fact met the standard, that he had rejected the standard, or he might be non-specific. A bold declaration that the standard had been met to the extent that any proof of 'sabotage' would be impossible, has some attractions. Any evidence which tended to prove his usage of such a mechanism would tend to disprove his having done so. He might, however, fall victim to the allegation that while his design was incompetent his attempt was effective through inadvertency.

A false statement that standard 6 had been considered but had *not* been implemented would be more protective, and although this could scarcely provide much public reassurance, it might be suggested that the denial was legally required and therefore not to be taken seriously. The third course is probably the most satisfactory, and it might be possible to make a non-specific reference to standard 6 in a manner which, by convention, might serve as reassurance that the protections afforded by the standard had not been ignored. It might be stated, for example, that 'the security provisions of system x are designed to meet the requirements of the Birmingham (1974) draft security standards for computer medical records, with the exception of standard 6 whose full implementation proved to be elusive'. It would have the additional advantage of being true.

Summary

The technical protection of computer medical records from unauthorized access can be reduced to the problems of encipherment and authorization. Secure encipherment can be accomplished by the appropriate use of non-constant keys generated jointly from within each record, from the record sequence number, from the file generation number and from authorization keys. Particular implementations are investigated as examples. A set of operational standards is derived and is offered for use as a reference standard.

Reference
FEISTAL, H. (1973). 'Cryptography and computer privacy', *Scientific American*, **228**, no. 5, 15–23.

Appendix 1
Specifications of subroutines **ENCODE, DECODE, and ENTRY**

```
SUBROUTINE ENCODE(KRECD,N,NUM,KEY,KSTEP)
DIMENSION KRECD(N)
DATA NE/0/
CALL ENTRY(N,NUM,KSTEP,NE)
KRECD(NE)= MOD2(KEY,KRECD(NE))
NB=N-I
DO 2 J=1,NB
NF=NE+KSTEP
IF(NF.GT.N) NF=NF-N
KRECD(NF)=MOD2(KRECD(NE),KRECD(NF))
2 NE=NF
NE=0
NF=0
NB=0
RETURN
END


SUBROUTINE ENTRY(N,NUM,KSTEP,NE)
K=KSTEP*2
NF=NUM+111
DO 2 U=1,K,3
2 NF=J*NE-J*NE/N*N+1
RETURN
END


SUBROUTINE DECODE(KRECD,N,NUM,KEY,KSTEP)
DIMENSION KRECD(N)
DATA NE/0/
CALL ENTRY(N,NUM,KSTEP,NE)
NB=N-I
NF=NE+(N-1)*KSTEP-1
NF=NF-NF/N*N+1
DO 2 J=1,NB
NE=NF-KSTEP
IF (NE.LT.1) NE=NE+N
KRECD(NF)=MOD2(KRECD(NE),KRECD(NF))
2 NF=NE
KRECD(NE)=MOD2(KEY,KRECD(NE))
RETURN
END
```

These subroutines operate jointly upon an integer array KRECD of size N understood to be a record read from, or to be written to, a data file. ENCODE and DECODE both call ENTRY which calculates the address within the record at which the encipherment/decipherment process begins. In particular applications, subroutine ENTRY may be altered or rewritten. For some purposes, DECODE and ENCODE may be used in a reverse sense.

Arguments KEY and KSTEP should contain respectively the authorization key and stepping frequency generated during the authorization process. The value NUM should be a reproduceable function of the record number within the file and of the file generation number.

In an ordinary updating operation KEY and KSTEP will be the same for the DECODE and the ENCODE operation, while NUM will change. Where authorizations and keys are reissued, KEY and KSTEP in the ENCODE operation will be altered.

Example of usage:

```
.
.
.
READ . . .
CALL DECODE (KRECD, N, KFILEA +KRECDA +KONST, KEYA, KSTEPA)
.
.
.
CALL ENCODE (KRECD, N, KFILEB +KRECDB +KONST, KEYB, KSTEPB)
WRITE . . .
.
.
.
```

Subroutines ENCODE and DECODE make use of the sub-program FUNCTION MOD2. It is envisaged that this subroutine is written in machine code or assembly code in a form which can be called by a higher-level language program.

Appendix 2
Specification of subroutine KEYS

```
      SUBROUTINE KEY (KBLOK,N,KEYA,KEYB,KSTEPA,KSTEPB,VALID)
      DIMENSION KBLOK (N)
      LOGICAL VALID,RESET
      DATA KEYZ/3H   /, KEYX/3HKEY/,  JZ/2/
      VALID=.TRUE.
      READ(1,1)JA,KEYA,KEYW,KEYC,KEYBR,KEYCR,JAR,KXR,KSTEPR,LOCK
    1 FORMAT(I3,5A3,3I3,A3)
      RESET=(KEYC.NE.KEYZ)
      JC=JA+2
      JD=JA+21
      JF=JA+JZ
      IF((JD+1).GT.N.OR.JF.GT.N) GOTO 30
      DO 20 J = JC,JD
      IF(KEYZ.EQ.MOD2(KEYW,KBLOK(J))) GO TO 20
      IF(KEYA.EQ.MOD2(KEYW,KBLOK(J))) GO TO 21
   20 CONTINUE
   30 KEYA=KEYZ
      KSTEPA=0
      IF(KEYC.EQ.KEYX) GO TO 40
      KEYB=KEYZ
      KSTEPB=0
      VALID=.FALSE.
      RETURN
   21 IF(RESET.AND.KEYC.NE.MOD2(KEYW,KBLOK(JD+1)    GO TO 30
      KSTEPA=MOD2(KEYW,KBLOK(JA+1))
      KSTEPB=KSTEPA
      KX=MOD2(KEYW,KBLOK(JA))
      KEYA=MOD2(KBLOK(JF),KBLOK(KX))
      KEYB=KEYA
      IF(.NOT.RESET) RETURN
COMMENT.   THIS TERMINATES NORMAL AUTHORIZATION PROCEDURE.
C          IDENTICAL READ/WRITE KEYS IN KEYA/KEYB AND KSTEPA/KSTEPB.
C          RESETTING PROCEDURE FOLLOWS AND RESULTS BOTH IN CHANGES T(
C          KBLOK AND ALTERATION OF THE WRITE-KEYS, KEYB AND KSTEPB.
   40 CONTINUE
      IF(JAR.LE.0.OR.KSTEPR.LE.0.OR.LOCK.EQ.KEYZ.OR.KXR.LE.0.OR.
     1KXR.GT.N)  GOTO 30
      JC=JAR+2
      JD=JAR+21
      JF=JAR+JZ
      IF((JD+1).GT.N.OR.JF.GT.N) GOTO 30
      KBLOK(JAR)=MOD2(KXR,KEYBR)
      KBLOK(JAR+1)=MOD2(KSTEPR,KEYBR)
      READ(1,2)(KBLOK(K),K=JC,JD)
    2 FORMAT(20A3)
      KBLOK(JD+1)=MOD2(KEYCR,KEYBR)
      KBLOK(KXR)=MOD2(KBLOK(JF),LOCK)
      DO 41 J=JC,JD
   41 KBLOK(J)=MOD2(KBLOK(J),KEYBR)
      KEYB=LOCK
      KSTEPB=KSTEPR
      RETURN
      END
```

Subroutine KEYS manipulates an authorization process in an integer array KBLOK of size N, understood as the header block of a data file. In normal use the whole of the header block will be stored in an enciphered form, for example through the use of ENCODE and DECODE. SUBROUTINE KEYS operations are performed on the deciphered versions and any encipherment/decipherment processes referred to below and performed by KEYS are at a secondary level. The SUB-ROUTINE offers two main facilities, the first relating to the normal authorization process and the second to resetting the authorization keys.

Example: CALL KEYS (KBLOK, N, KEYA, KEYB, KSTEPA, KSTEPB, VALID)

A. The authorization process depends upon an input key card the contents of which are used to decipher a part of the header block, relate a key on the card to a key in the header block, and if there is a valid match, to generate keys for the decipherment of all subsequent records on the file. This key card uses three fields, each of three columns, the fields being numbered and named as follows:

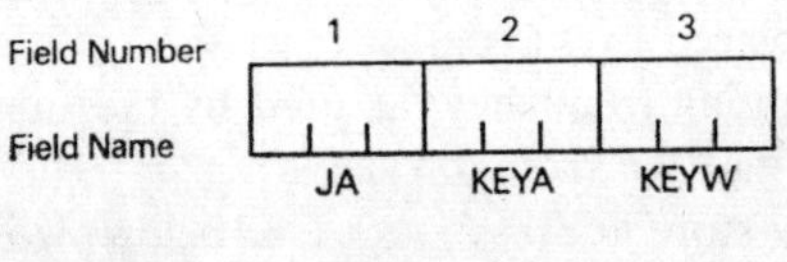

Example: b27AAZQQQ

In this example 27 is a reference address in the header file and QQQ is a decipherment key which uncovers an area of header block related to this address. A match for AAZ is sought within this area. Following a successful match the logical variable VALID is set TRUE; otherwise FALSE.

Following a valid exit KEYA = KEYB = the value KEY required by ENCODE and DECODE; also KSTEPA = KSTEPB = the stepping frequency KSTEP required by ENCODE and DECODE. The use of KEYS may be followed by extraction of a 'file-generation' number from the header block of the input tape, its modification and recording in the header block of the output tape, and the use of the old and the new values in the arguments NUM required by subroutines DECODE and ENCODE.

B. The setting and resetting procedures involve the use of subsequent fields in the authorization card, numbered and named as follows:

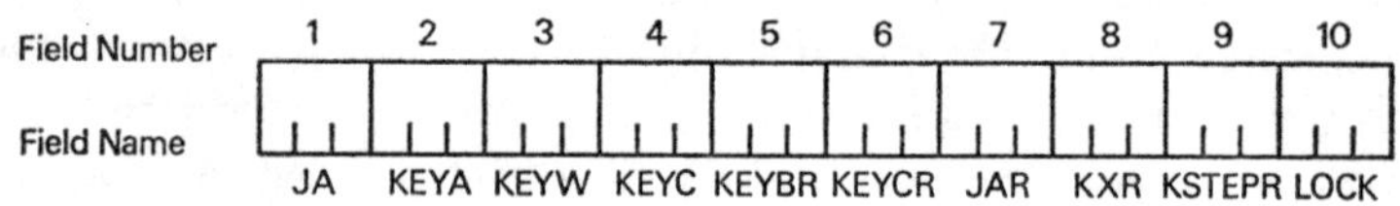

Example: b27AAZQQQPPPRRRSSSb20b49b13NNN . . . plus a second
card with up to 20 three-character authorization keys.

The additional operations are triggered by a non-blank value in KEYC (field 4). Normal validation, and the construction of keys for deciphering the input file, is followed by reconstruction of the header block to produce a new cipher system for the output file, this process depending upon a successful match between KEYC and the old value stored in the header block. Successful matching is followed by:

1. Reading another card containing a set of up to 20 authorization keys against which ordinary users will have to match their issued authorization (eg AAZ above).

2. JA is replaced by JAR.

3. KEYW is replaced by KEYBR.

4. KEYC is replaced by KEYCR.

5. A new stepping frequency, as used by the subroutines ENCODE and DECODE, is inserted from KSTEPR.

6. A new 'key-store address', KXR (see below) is inserted.

7. A new locking key, LOCK, is introduced to the header block.

C. Initial settings are catered for by a facility responding to the characters KEY in field 4. This is a 'master' facility in that it can always be used to reset output keys and bypasses the need to match the first three fields correctly, but it does not give access to the input file and could not be used by a thief. For specific applications the contents of this initial 'key' can be set through the data statement near the head of the subroutine.

Example: bbbbbbbbbbKEYRRRSSSb20b49b13NNN . . . plus a second
card with up to 20 authorization keys.

D. Header block layout.

		JA	JA+2					
		KX	STEP	AA G	AA H	AA I	AA J	AA K
AA L	AA M	AA N	AA O	AA P	AA Q	AA R	AA S	AA T
						JA+22		
AA U	AA V	AA W	AA X	AA Y	AA Z	KEYC		
				KX				
				ZZZ				

The reference address in KBLOK is JA and this address holds the 'key store address' KX. The next address holds the decipherment 'step-parameter', KSTEP, used by ENCODE and DECODE and the next twenty addresses hold alternative authorization keys. Following this is the guardian key, KEYC. All locations JA to JA$+22$ are enciphered by KEYW.

The record-closure KEY required by ENCODE and DECODE is reset from the input variable LOCK. The value is not actually stored anywhere but is reconstructed from the value held in location KX. This value is constructed in the first place on the basis of a MOD2 addition between LOCK and the contents of location (JA$+2$). It is reconstructed in the same manner.

E. A successful authorization resetting procedure is terminated with VALID set TRUE. However, this setting does not guarantee that the procedure has been successfully completed and there are several pathways through which VALID may be set TRUE in the presence of nonsense keys.

List of papers from the Health Services Research Centre, University of Birmingham

Brennan, Mary, E., and Knox, E. G. (1973). 'An investigation into the purposes, accuracy and effective uses of the blind register in England', *Br. J. prev. soc. Med.* **27,** 154.

—— and Opit, L. J. (1973). 'The demand for family planning advice amongst patients in a district maternity hospital', *Br. med. J.* **3,** 19.

—— —— (1974). 'The unwanted birth', *J. Biosoc. Sci.* **6,** 407.

Brown, E. L., and Knox, E. G. (1972). 'Epidemiological approach to Parkinson's Disease', *Lancet*, **i,** 974.

Cross, K. W., and Farmer, R. D. T. (1975). 'Influenza vaccine in the elderly', *Community Hlth*, **6,** 224.

Cumming, G., and Goldsmith, O. (1971). 'Inclined planes or cogwheels', in McLachlan, G. (ed.), *In Low Gear?*, pp. 55–97, Occasional Hundreds 2 (Oxford University Press for the Nuffield Provincial Hospitals Trust).

Farmer, R. D. T., and Cross, K. W. (1973). 'The National Health Service number', *Br. J. prev. soc. Med.* **27,** 53.

—— Knox, E. G., Cross, K. W., and Crombie, D. L. (1974). 'Executive council lists and general practitioner files', ibid. **28,** 49.

—— (1974). 'Community care—a model system', *Internat J. Nurs. Stud.* **11,** 21.

—— and Harvey, P. G. (1974). 'Alienated youth—a preliminary study of a group of rootless young people—social and personality characteristics', *Soc. Sci. & Med.* **88,** 191.

Goldsmith, O. (1972). 'Medical and non-medical administration', *Br. Hosp. J. and Soc. Serv. Rev.* **82,** 606.

—— (1972). 'Organisation of medical work in hospital', ibid. **82,** 2171.

—— (1973). 'The implementation of research: an administrative view', *Hosp. Hlth Serv. Rev.* 125.

Holland, W. W., and Knox, E. G. (1974). Introduction to 'Research in Medical Care', *Br. med. Bull.* **30,** 195.

Hood, J. E., and Farmer, R. D. T. (1974). 'A comparative study of frequent and infrequent attenders at a general practice', *Internat. J. Nurs. Stud.* **11**, 147.

Knox, E. G., and Mahon, D. F. (1970). 'Evaluation of infant at risk registers', *Arch. Dis. Childh.* **45**, 634.

—— (1970). 'Problems in health service computing applications' in Abrams, M. E. (ed.), *Medical Computing—Progress and Problems*, p. 353 (London: Chatto and Windus).

—— (1970). 'Strategies of medical computing. Some comments on two new books', *Meth. Inform. Med.* **9**, 187.

—— (1971). 'Quantification in medicine. A case for the computer', *Times Lit. Suppl.* (3 September), pp. 1059–60.

—— (1972). 'Anencephalus and dietary intakes', *Br. J. prev. soc. Med.* **26**, 219.

—— Morris, J. N., and Holland, W. W. (1972). 'Planning medical information systems in a unified health service', *Lancet*, **ii**, 696.

—— (1973). 'Computer simulations of cervical cytology screening programmes', McLachlan, G. (ed.), *The Future—and Present Indicatives, Problems and Progress in Medical Care*, Ninth Series (Oxford University Press for the Nuffield Provincial Hospitals Trust).

—— (1973). 'Computer simulations of industrial hazards', *Br. J. indust. Med.* **30**, 54.

—— (1973). 'Diet and ischaemic heart disease', *Lancet*, **i**, 1465.

—— (1974). 'Twins and neural tube defects', *Br. J. prev. soc. Med.* **28**, 73.

—— (1974). 'Multiphasic screening', *Lancet*, **ii**, 39.

—— (1974). 'New etiologies for ischaemic heart disease', *Am. Heart J.* **88**, 809.

—— (1975). 'Computer simulation studies of alternative population screening policies', in Bailey, N. T. J., and Thompson, M. (eds), *Systems Aspects of Health Planning*, pp. 191–201 (Vienna: International Institute for Applied Systems Analysis).

McKeown, T., Cross, K. W., and Keating, D. N. (1971). 'The influence of hospital siting on patient visiting', *Lancet*, **ii**, 1082.

Opit, L. J. (1972) 'Long range planning for what?', in Abrams, M. E, (ed.), *Spectrum 1971*, pp. 173–81 (London: Butterworths).

—— and Cross, K. W. (1973). 'Comparing hospital costs', *Hospital*, **69**, 44.

—— —— (1973). 'A model for comparing clinical salaries in acute hospital services', ibid. **69,** 254.

—— —— (1973). 'Strategy for allocating revenue to medical services', *Br. med. J.* **4,** 13.

—— and GREENHILL, D. (1974). 'Prevalence of gallstones in relation to differing treatment rates for biliary disease', *Br. J. prev. soc. Med.* **28,** 268.

—— and BRENNAN, MARY E. (1974). 'The demand for surgical sterilisation amongst patients in a district maternity hospital', ibid. **28,** 19.

—— and FARMER, R. D. T. (1974). 'Cost of dispensing in the pharmaceutical services', *Lancet,* **i,** 190.

RHYS HEARN, C. (1973). 'Evaluation of patients' nursing needs: prediction of staffing', in McLachlan, G. (ed.), *The Future—and Present Indicatives, Problems and Progress in Medical Care*, Ninth Series (Oxford University Press for the Nuffield Provincial Hospitals Trust).

—— and YOUNG, D. (1975). 'A problem-oriented management scheme', *Meth. Inform. Med.* **14,** 13.